ADVANCING
RELATIONSHIP-BASED
CULTURES

MARY KOLOROUTIS, RN
DAVID ABELSON, MD
EDITORS

ADVANCING RELATIONSHIP-BASED CULTURES
Copyright © 2017 by Creative Health Care Management

Library of Congress Cataloging-in-Publication Data
Softcover ISBN 13: 978-1-886624-97-9
ebook ISBN 13: 978-1-886624-98-6

Printed and bound in the United States of America.

21 20 19 18 17   5 4 3 2 1

First Printing: May 2017

Library of Congress Cataloging-in-Publication Data

Names: Koloroutis, Mary, editor. | Abelson, David, editor. | Creative Health Care
Management (Minneapolis, Minn.), issuing body.

Title: Advancing relationship-based cultures / edited by Mary Koloroutis, David Abelson.

Description: Minneapolis, MN : Creative Health Care Management, [2017] | Includes
bibliographical references and index.

Identifiers: LCCN 2017013285 (print) | LCCN 2017014410 (ebook) | ISBN 9781886624986 |
ISBN 9781886624979 (pbk. : alk. paper) | ISBN 9781886624986 (ebook)

Subjects: | MESH: Professional-Patient Relations | Professional-Family Relations |
Interprofessional Relations | Organizational Culture | Self-care | Empathy

Classification: LCC R727.3 (ebook) | LCC R727.3 (print) | NLM W 62 | DDC 610.69--dc23

LC record available at https://lccn.loc.gov/2017013285

Cover and interior design by James Monroe Design, LLC.

CREATIVE
HEALTH CARE
MANAGEMENT

For permission and ordering information, write to:
Creative Health Care Management, Inc.
6200 Baker Road, Suite 200
Minneapolis, MN 55346

www.chcm.com
800.728.7766 / 952.854.9015

CONTENTS

SECTION THREE: TEAMWORK AND INTERPROFESSIONAL PRACTICE

SECTION FOUR: PATIENT CARE DELIVERY AND SYSTEMS THINKING

SECTION FIVE: EVIDENCE

APPENDIXES

FOREWORD

The Giver and the Receiver Are One

DR. ROBIN YOUNGSON, COFOUNDER OF HEARTS IN HEALTHCARE

In our Hearts in Healthcare workshops, small groups of nurses, therapists, and doctors sit in a circle sharing stories of extraordinary connection with their patients. We hold a sacred space by bringing attention to our breath and allowing the room to become very still. Only the person holding the heart-shaped "talking stone" is allowed to speak, so we place the stone in the center of the circle and wait in silence for each person to take the stone.

In one workshop, a nurse stepped forward to pick up the stone. Sitting quietly, she clutched the stone to her breast, doubled over, and wept for some minutes. Every person in the room cried with her. Not a word was said. She was weeping with the pain of working in a health care system that for so many years had not given her permission to care and heal in the way her heart desired. She also wept for the sheer joy of those times she had overcome the limitations of the system to make the compassionate connection anyway.

When she eventually spoke, she didn't share a story; she just offered seven words: "The giver and the receiver are one." In that sacred moment, everybody understood her meaning. She was talking about the very foundation of the healing connection.

In the sacred circle, we've heard many stories of profound healing. It begins with the capacity of a practitioner to go with patients to their darkest places, to sit with them in despair and loss, and not flinch. Health care affords us countless opportunities to heal ourselves and our colleagues, as we work together to heal our patients and their families. What makes this multifaceted healing necessary is our common human wound, and what makes this healing *possible* is our willingness and ability to forge healthy relationships.

Because the giver and receiver are one, when we extend compassion, our own compassionate heart expands. If we want to change the health care system, we first have to change ourselves. We have to work on healing our own wounds, practice self-compassion, let go of harshness and judgment, and develop a sensitive awareness of our way of being. As a doctor, I have to ask myself, "What is the spirit I bring to every patient encounter?"

In my daily work as an anesthesiologist, I try to meet each patient as a human being first, to put them at ease, to connect to their everyday life. I make sure I'm not standing over my patients, which is always intimidating. I make myself very still for a moment before I ask the patient, "How are you?" My manner makes clear that this is not a throwaway social greeting; I mean it. I love this moment of connection. I watch intently with all my senses ready to receive. I know that almost every patient is anxious or frightened, so I'm looking closely for signs of tension. I find out their fears and concerns, and I validate their feelings. Every day, during moments like these, I learn things that are truly important for my clinical care.

I take the time to do this with every patient who comes to the OR, no matter how busy I am. I find that it ultimately saves an enormous amount of time. My cases go better, the complications are fewer, the patients recover more quickly, their side effects are lessened, and I have a more rewarding day, made invaluable by the joy of human connection.

If we want to make health care more compassionate and to strengthen relationships, we have to be the compassionate healer to the system; we need to stop trying to fix what's wrong with the system and strengthen what's right. So it's with satisfaction that I see this wonderful book on relationship-based cultures consider every level of the system, from the intimate details of individual patient care to issues of leadership and culture. No other approach will make a difference.

The giver and the receiver truly are one: Every time we bring compassion to the work we do, we advance a relationship-based culture, and we move closer to achieving a health care system we can be proud to leave to the next generations.

DR. ROBIN YOUNGSON IS THE CO-FOUNDER OF HEARTS IN HEALTHCARE AND THE AUTHOR OF *TIME TO CARE: HOW TO LOVE YOUR PATIENTS AND YOUR JOB* AND *FROM HERO TO HEALER: AWAKENING THE INNER ACTIVIST.*

A Note about the Use of Gender Pronouns

Throughout this book, we alternate masculine and feminine pronouns more or less equally in instances where the individual could be any gender. While this method of inclusive language is imperfect, we have used it whenever possible instead of the singular *they*.

I think health care is more about love than about most other things. If there isn't at the core of this two human beings who have agreed to be in a relationship where one is trying to help relieve the suffering of another, which is love, you can't get to the right answer here.

Donald Berwick

OVERVIEW

Advancing Relationship-Based Cultures

MARY KOLOROUTIS AND DAVID ABELSON

The premise of *Advancing Relationship-Based Cultures* is simple. Given that relationships permeate every atom of health care, it follows quite naturally that everything in health care will work better when relationships are healthy. Medical miracles, alleviated suffering, and enhanced comfort all take place between human beings. They take place when human beings who are suffering enter the sphere of a group of human beings who are as committed to caring for them as whole, complex people as they are committed to applying their technical skill and knowledge to the healing of their physical ailments.

All of the technical aspects of health care occur in the context of human relationships, which means that all of the technical tasks underlying the provision of care work better when we tend to relationships. Discernment and decisions, in the face of complexity and uncertainty, improve when professionals collaborate. Just as jets crash when cockpit teams lack the interpersonal trust to speak up, patients die when health care team members don't feel the psychological safety and interpersonal trust to speak up.

The inseparability of tasks and processes from people begins to answer the question of why we chose the term *relationship-based culture*. Although we recognize that care, safety, quality, and financial health emerge from tasks *and* relationships, we also know that health care is currently tilted toward an emphasis on tasks at the expense of relationships.

Our intent is to restore the balance. The key is to be relationship-based, while being process-focused.

The Impact of Healthy Relationships

It is easy to make the case for the importance of healthy relationships in health care. What has traditionally been much harder is to delve deeply into the how-to. How are healthy relationships formed? What seems always to be present when relationships are healthy and productive? What is missing when relationships are troubled or fractured?

A theme that will permeate this book is: Healthy relationships are formed when people consistently *attune* to one another, *wonder* with and about one another, *follow* the cues provided by one another, and *hold* one another with respect and dignity. The book *See Me as a Person: Creating Therapeutic Relationships with Patients and their Families* (Koloroutis & Trout, 2012) explains how clinicians can create therapeutic relationships with patients and families using the therapeutic practices of attuning, wondering, following, and holding. *Advancing Relationship-Based Cultures* is, in part, about the application of those same practices to all relationships at all levels and in all disciplines in order to improve every relationship in an organization.

Healthy relationships are formed when people consistently attune to one another, wonder with and about one another, follow the cues provided by one another, and hold one another with respect and dignity.

Note that we used the term *advancing* rather than *creating* in the title of this book. We know that you are not creating relationship-based cultures from scratch because healthy productive relationships are already a part of your care, teamwork, leadership, and your culture as a whole. In fact, we are certain that they are part of it because the four therapeutic practices (which we will refer to as *relational practices* when used outside of the therapeutic relationship) were discovered through an analysis of healthy relationships in health care settings—in other words, through an analysis of the best moments of people like you in organizations much like your own. You and everyone in your organization attune, wonder, follow, and hold in your best moments. One of the aims of this book is to help make the four relational practices the norm for each person in your organization.

Systems Thinking and Systems Design for Relationship-Based Cultures

Modern health care occurs within complex systems of people, processes, and structures. Everything we aspire to accomplish in health care arises from how people, processes, and structures relate to one another.

Here's how systems thinking applies to an analysis of culture: There is no discrete part of an organizational system called *culture* that can be isolated and fine-tuned. Instead, culture *emerges* as patterns of interactions between people, processes, and structures. Given that culture is generally expressed through patterns of conversation and behavior—the "people" portion of systems—it is easy to think of culture as arising only from the people dimension.

> *Culture emerges as patterns of interactions between people, processes, and structures.*

A simple example, though, demonstrates the degree to which culture emerges from how people, processes, and structures interact. Consider walking into a primary care clinic. If you walk into enough clinics, you will develop within minutes a visceral sense of how welcoming the culture is. The obvious indicator will be the receptionist greeting you without delay, with a warm smile, and with direct eye contact, rather than remaining buried in the computer and, without looking up, asking you to verify your name and birth date.

That's the people portion of the equation, but let's look at the impact of structure on how welcomed you feel. Does the clinic's structure feel dark? Does a directory, rather than a human being, greet you? What about the ease of parking or using public transportation? How does the décor make you feel? Does it jangle your nerves, or does it soothe you? Is the environment noisy (perhaps a TV is loud) or peaceful? Consider how the soothing-rather-than-jangly environment will impact not just your mood but also the mood of the receptionist and how he greets you.

Now let's look at the impact of process on a welcoming culture. How easy was it to make an appointment for your clinic visit? Did you do it rapidly online, or did you walk in grumpy and without an appointment because the phone waits were interminable? Are follow-up appointments made in the examination room, or are patients asked to go to the front desk to make a return appointment, forcing the receptionist to multitask and make follow-up appointments as well as greet patients checking in? Processes that do not work well stress team members, contribute to burn-out, and interfere with the team's ability to warmly welcome and interact with patients.

Now add the interaction of management processes with people and structure. Was the receptionist who greeted you hired with cultural fit in mind? What orientation to the value of patient relationships was pro-vided for her? Does the operating rhythm of the clinic include convening the entire team weekly to tell stories about when welcoming went well and to ask the people closest to the work how things can go better? Or does the team convene far less frequently—perhaps only once a year—to talk about changes that are being "rolled out"?

Consider now the likelihood of a welcoming culture emerging in which people work in a quiet, soothing environment using processes that support them, in which their input on process improvement is valued, as opposed to one emerging from a system in which people work in a noisy, nerve-jangling environment using processes that do not work well for them or for patients, and who rarely (or never) meet as a team to consider how to improve.

This example demonstrates how people, processes, and structures interact to create a more welcoming or less welcoming culture. The same sorts of interactions are relevant to all aspects of culture. Thus, the work of advancing a relationship-based culture requires work on all three com-ponent parts—people, processes, and structures.

In the workplace, people tend to affiliate with the individuals with whom they work most closely on a day-to-day basis and/or with groups with whom they identify, such as other members of their profession, dis-cipline, or work group. Subcultures emerge from these affiliated groups, and these subcultures typically have distinct characteristics. In fact, vis-itors to the team may discern the subculture and its general impression within minutes. Because of this fact of life, it is easy to slip back into thinking that the culture of an organization is entirely the domain of the people portion of the system.

It's not true, though. All three components of the system—people, processes, and structures—create the culture of your organization. Patients and families experience your organization through your culture. Attuned, compassionate teams can go a long way toward creating a welcoming culture, but if the processes and structures create barriers to team members being attuned and compassionate, patients and their families are still going to end up feeling dropped.

This book, while focusing most often on the people portion of the equation, also addresses the processes and structures that can and must contribute to the ability of all people in health care to provide attuned, compassionate care. One of our assumptions is that ideal care begins with individual self-awareness on the part of each clinician or caregiver. Another is that all processes and structures can and must be designed to be as supportive as possible of each caregiver's ability to connect meaningfully with each other and with patients and their families.

All processes and structures can and must be designed to be as supportive as possible of each caregiver's ability to connect meaningfully with each other and with patients and their families.

This is why systems thinking must inform system design. With a clear vision of what we want to see emerge from the system as a whole (as well as from every system within the system), we consider the interaction of all of the people, processes, and structures involved. If our vision is for every patient, every family member, every team member, and every individual in our organizations to feel seen, appreciated, and held, we will keep that vision clearly in mind when we think about and design our systems.

Relationship-Based Care

Relationship-Based Care (RBC) is a philosophy, a way of being, and an operational blueprint (Koloroutis, 2004). Since Creative Health Care Management published the book *Relationship-Based Care: A Model for Transforming Practice* in 2004, thousands of health care leaders are putting RBC into action and cultivating positive and healing organizations. Such leaders work with the understanding that people actively advance their culture when they share a common purpose and vision; when they are inspired and supported to take ownership for living the vision; when infrastructure is designed to support new ways of working; when there is an investment in education and learning; and when visible evidence of success is shared widely, which in turn inspires further commitment and improvement (Felgen, 2007).

While the book *Relationship-Based Care* provides an in-depth look into RBC as a philosophy and operational blueprint, this book focuses on what it takes to truly advance the relational components of RBC into a vital and healing culture.

The Three Key Relationships in RBC

Relationship-Based Care posits that three key relationships have a profound influence on culture: relationship with self, relationships with team members, and relationships with patients and families (Koloroutis, 2004, pp. 5–6). Note the order here: relationship with self is first, followed by relationships with teammates, and finally, relationships with patients and families. We use this order not to signal priority but to acknowledge that certain relationships depend on others. Healthy, trusting team relationships, for example, are dependent on how the individuals involved relate to themselves—how self-aware people are and how able they are to manage their behavior and emotions. Healthy relationships with patients and families are dependent on the relationships that individuals have both with themselves and with their teams.

In our work with organizations throughout the world that are using RBC as their care model, this is one of the concepts that consistently resonates most strongly with people at all levels in the organization. They can see immediately the practicality of self-care and healthy teams, as well as how they directly affect patient care. The quality of the three key relationships also, of course, has a profound effect on the emerging culture.

Think of the people portion of an organization as a chemical compound. In a huge organization, it may be hard to perceive the difference when one person is added or another is removed, but each time there is a personnel change, the compound itself—the organization—changes. It is also true that when the existing group of people advances in some way, or suffers a loss, the organization changes. We've already asserted that this is why relationships matter, but it also happens to be the reason any given individual's way of being matters. People who are stretched and stressed make the organizational culture more stretched and more stressed. People who find ways to take care of themselves while they take care of others make the organizational culture more caring.

RBC's three key relationships will be revisited throughout this book.

The Eight Dimensions of the RBC Model as a Framework for This Book

This book advocates RBC as the operational model of choice, as do (we assume) a large segment of our readers. For the ease of readers who are already familiar with RBC and to help illustrate how every dimension of RBC is optimized when all relationships are improved, we have organized the chapters of this book according to the dimensions of the model. What follows is a glimpse into the organizational framework of this book, along with brief descriptions of each chapter.

Section One
Healing Cultures/Patients and Families in the Center of Care

A healing culture is both the inspirational vision and the ultimate outcome for Relationship-Based Care. Healing cultures hold all people with respect and dignity and cultivate relationships and norms that help people to realize their full potential.

Healing cultures hold all people with respect and dignity and cultivate relationships and norms that help people to realize their full potential.

One of the keys to a healing culture is to hold patients and families at the center of all we do. Our obligation to provide the best possible care within a continuously improving health care culture means we must provide inspiring and supportive leadership and cultivate high-performing teams, exquisite care delivery design, and healthy relationships.

When we use the word *patient*, it is to be understood that we are including residents, clients, and all others using health-related services. There has been much discussion in recent years about the use of the word *patient* in a world where many of the people seeking health care services are neither ill nor injured. We respect the discussion and even the disagreement; the word is imperfect. One thing the word *patient* accomplishes quite well, however, is that it distinguishes people seeking care and health-related service from customers or consumers. Patients, even if they are well, are people seeking care or improved wellness. Patients who are ill are experiencing vulnerability and suffering. Conversely, customers and consumers are people who purchase goods or services and whose business we want to attract and retain. While there can be some overlap among these two groups, we believe that this is a key distinction, and that health systems designed with patients and families in mind will be consistently superior to health systems designed for customers and consumers.

Chapter One explains the four basic relational practices that improve the quality of all relationships while optimizing the personal authenticity of every person who uses them. In the book *See Me as a Person,* Mary Koloroutis and Michael Trout identified the therapeutic practices of attuning, wondering, following, and holding as the building blocks of all therapeutic relationships. While *See Me as a Person* refers to attuning, wondering, following, and holding as *therapeutic practices,* they acknowledge that these practices are present in *all* effective, meaningful relationships.

Because this book on advancing relationship-based cultures is to some extent a how-to guide for nurturing and improving relationships, we have chosen to emphasize the importance of actively recognizing and engaging in these practices, not just with patients and families but with everyone in our organizations and in our relationships with ourselves. When even one of us chooses to attune, wonder, follow, and hold, relationships—and therefore cultures—improve.

In **Chapter Two**, Brett Long and Rebecca Smith show how attuning, wondering, following, and holding can be used in one's relationship with self. The only real hope for creating healing cultures in our health care environments rests in the possibility that each person in health care can cultivate a healing culture within him- or herself. It is possible that the most effective, sustainable way to create change "out there" is to create exactly the change you'd like to see in the world, right in your own mind, your own heart, your own practice, your own home, your own life.

> *When even one of us chooses to attune, wonder, follow, and hold, relationships—and therefore cultures—improve.*

In **Chapter Three**, Mary Koloroutis and Michael Trout introduce the provocative notion that most people seeking care are in a *non-ordinary state.* Their vulnerability is heightened, and along with it, their need for human connection. Once we are aware of this non-ordinary state and the heightened need for attuned human connection that goes with it, we have an ethical choice to make. Do we use the therapeutic tool of attunement and connect with those in our care? Or is it acceptable to forgo attunement and just get on with our tasks?

In **Chapter Four**, Mary Koloroutis, Marky Medeiros, and Mary Griffin Strom provide a look directly into the thoughts and feelings of the family members of patients. Can we reasonably consider a health care culture "healing" if it does not tend to the needs of our patients' loved ones? This chapter explores how negative perceptions of family members are formed and perpetuated. It also invites greater understanding and the potential for greater acceptance and support by lifting up and listening to the voices of families who teach us what matters most to them and their loved ones. The beauty in their lessons is that the things the families of our patients want most do not result in more work for caregivers. Readers will discover that what matters most to the families of our patients are the simple things.

Section Two
Leadership

Leadership sets the tone for an entire organization. Leaders in cultures that embrace Relationship-Based Care as their organizational model are poised to make a major impact, no matter what their role or level of influence. When the entire organization is focused on improving relationships, leaders have a heightened opportunity to be more overtly relational. In relationship-based cultures, vulnerability, humility, authenticity, and transparency are not seen as weaknesses; instead they contribute to a deep sense that we are, indeed, all in this together.

In relationship-based cultures, vulnerability, humility, authenticity, and transparency are not seen as weaknesses; instead they contribute to a deep sense that we are all in this together.

In **Chapter Five**, Jayne Felgen and Pamela Schaid show us how a relationship-based culture is advanced when leaders love the people they work with and love the work they do. While *love* has not been a word traditionally associated with work and business, that seems to be changing, not only in the world of health care but in the world of business overall. As we have been privileged to work with health care leaders through the years, we have discovered that, among those who enjoy the greatest success and job satisfaction, a thread of love permeates their leadership and their cultures. This chapter is the result of its authors talking with eight leaders they identified as *loving leaders*.

In **Chapter Six**, David Abelson looks at the role of physicians in advancing the cultures of organizations. Based on the idea that "with great power comes great responsibility," this chapter examines the power physicians have, by virtue of their role, to influence culture for better or worse and outlines small actions physicians can take that result in a profound positive difference in the cultures of the organizations and departments in which they work. This chapter proposes the provocative idea that advancing a relationship-based culture benefits physicians as much as it benefits anyone else, including patients and families.

In **Chapter Seven**, Kristen Lombard, Donna Wright, and Tara Nichols introduce the notion of *relational competence* as a learnable, measurable set of skills, no less essential than technical competence. These authors share how relational competence can be embedded into an organization via its competency assessment process.

In **Chapter Eight**, Brett Long, Donna Wright, and Ann Flanagan Petry explain the strategic role that human resources (HR) leaders and departments can and must play in shaping the culture of the organization by embedding relational practices into the culture in every facet of the human resources function. In organizations in which the HR department is meeting its full potential, that department becomes a key player in making sure all of the organization's "people practices" are aligned with the broader goal of creating a high-performing enterprise.

Section Three
Teamwork and Interprofessional Practice

A discussion of teamwork and interprofessional practice in health care is inseparable from a discussion of the overall culture of an organization. In a world in which the borders between teams are becoming more and more flexible, people must be able to collaborate with people they don't know and who may do very different work. When people cannot rely on the advantage of knowing their team members well, relational skills are more valuable than ever.

In **Chapter Nine**, the interprofessional team of Donna Wright, Ann Flanagan Petry, Kary Gillenwaters, and David Abelson (a nurse, social worker, occupational therapist, and physician, respectively) describe what healthy interprofessional teaming looks like in practice. Healthy cultures are advanced when team members remember that their shared purpose is to promote the healing and wellbeing of patients and their loved ones. This chapter explores what healthy interprofessional teaming looks like when attuning, wondering, following, and holding are standard practices among team members.

Section Four
Patient Care Delivery and Systems Design

While we literally wrote the book on patient care delivery in inpatient settings (Koloroutis, 2004; Koloroutis, Felgen, Person, & Wessel, 2007; Manthey, 1980, 2002; Wessel & Manthey, 2015), *this* book addresses care delivery system design in all settings. It has been exhilarating to work through what it takes to bring to all of health care the time-tested principles of care that have helped patients and families in inpatient settings to feel held in our care for almost five decades.

In **Chapter Ten**, Susan Wessel, David Abelson, and Marie Manthey provide a comprehensive look at the principles and practices essential to designing care delivery systems, for use in all settings, that are truly relationship-based. While applying systems thinking to care delivery design, this chapter reveals the importance not merely of individuals within the system being attuned to patients, families, and one another but of the system itself being designed to promote a high level of attunement in all of the people it comprises.

Section Five
Evidence

Evidence is an available body of research and information indicating whether a pursuit (such as RBC) is effective. Evidence supporting the effectiveness of Relationship-Based Care is found in studies of effective leadership, communication, teamwork, quality and safety, emotional and social intelligence, compassion and love, positive organizational development, employee engagement, the patient experience, and the stories of our own RBC clients' success. We are pleased to share the evidence base on which RBC sits, as well as the ways in which RBC organizations have a distinct advantage when pursuing national recognitions, such as Magnet®* designation.

In **Chapter Eleven**, Ann Flanagan Petry, Susan Wessel, and Catherine Perrizo provide evidence that advancing cultures in which patients and

---

* MAGNET®, Magnet Recognition Program®, ANCC®, Magnet®, and the Journey to Magnet Excellence® are registered trademarks of the American Nurses Credentialing Center. The products and services of Creative Health Care Management are neither sponsored nor endorsed by ANCC. All rights reserved.

families are held at the center of care does in fact lead to improved outcomes. Leaders who have used RBC as an operational framework report positive outcomes in patient safety, quality, and experience; employee engagement and satisfaction; and financial performance. In work cultures in which people are given the tools and empowerment to take excellent care of themselves, one another, and the patients and families they serve, the overall performance of the organization improves.

In **Chapter Twelve,** Gen Guanci and Marky Medeiros show how success on a Relationship-Based Care journey can position an organization to pursue Magnet designation or other national recognitions and awards. Organizations that have used RBC as their operational model are likely to have established many of the structures, processes, and outcomes foundational to a successful Magnet journey.

The Language of Our Cultural Narratives

The language that pervades an organization cannot help but shape its culture. As we live our lives, we also continually "tell stories" about our lives, even though we don't always share our narratives with others. Because our individual stories play such a big part in our lives, it's quite possible that we create our life experiences just as much by what we say as by what we do (Smith, 2016). Within the context of an industry as vital as health care, this begs a very important question: Just how careful are we in how we talk about our work?

The acceptance or rejection of positive expressions of the meaning and purpose of our work matters to a culture. It matters a lot.

How often do we speak about our work with deep reverence for the everyday miracles we facilitate? And just as importantly, how acceptable is it, in your current culture, to express reverence? If you spoke with reverence about how honored you are to do the work you do, would your declaration be met with looks of respectful recognition, or would people roll their eyes and tell you to stop being so dramatic? The acceptance or rejection of positive expressions of the meaning and purpose of our work matters to a culture. It matters a lot.

In a keynote address at one of Creative Health Care Management's International Relationship-Based Care Symposia, best-selling author and acclaimed speaker Brené Brown talked about the importance of advancing a culture in which it's "cool to care." Within a culture in which people are feeling unseen and invalidated, it's very hard to be the lone person who stays positive and openly expresses the meaning and purpose of our work. As we think through the many disparaging labels a person of that sort might be saddled with, they are all a far cry from the most appropriate label we can think of: courageous. It takes a great deal of courage to stay both inwardly and outwardly positive in a culture in which people are dissatisfied and hurting. Interestingly, however, we find that it can take no small measure of courage to stay both inwardly and outwardly positive even in much healthier cultures.

We invite you to start noticing the language that is pervasive in your work environment. What words and phrases, positive or negative, do you hear people use most often? Are there phrases that rankle you every time you hear them? And what language do *you* use that, once you think about it, might not be actively advancing a healthier culture? Do you use war metaphors to speak about staff members who are on the "front lines" or about putting "boots on the ground" in a new department or clinic? Do you refer to people who are enthusiastic about a new initiative as having "drunk the Kool-Aid"—perhaps forgetting that that phrase refers to a group of people who in 1978, while brainwashed by a despotic cult leader, willingly killed themselves and their children by drinking cyanide-laced punch? Tremendous violence is hiding in some of our everyday language, and all of it matters because on some level we take it all in, whether we consciously notice it or not.

Now consider what phrases you say or hear that appeal to you as beautiful expressions of the meaning and purpose of a life devoted to the healing and wellbeing of patients and their families. We invite you to begin making an informal study of what language you would banish from your organization if you had the power to, and what language you would like to hear more often.

Because this is essentially a book about optimizing cultures through optimizing relationships, the thread that will carry most pervasively through the rest of this book is one that amplifies the four relational practices: attuning, wondering, following, and holding (Koloroutis & Trout, 2012). We believe that no prescribed language—no scripting— can improve relationships; rather, these four relational practices, which will be explained fully in Chapter One, put people into a mindset from which peaceful language is far more likely to flow. As you visit the chapters of this book, you'll have repeated opportunities to understand how every dimension of health care can be improved through the improvement of every relationship, and how every relationship cannot help but be improved by any person at any time, attuning, wondering, following, and holding.

Summary of Key Thoughts

- Since relationships permeate every atom of health care, everything in health care will work better when relationships are healthy.

- The four *therapeutic practices* are attuning, wondering, following, and holding. When we talk about them outside the context of the therapeutic relationship, they are referred to as *relational practices.*

- Healthy relationships are formed when people consistently attune to one another, wonder with and about one another, follow the cues provided by one another, and hold one another with respect and dignity.

- Culture is the result of interactions among people, processes, and structures. People, processes, and structures must all be addressed if a culture is to be advanced.

- Relationship-Based Care (RBC) is the organizational model that most directly advances relationship-based cultures.

- RBC posits that three key relationships have a profound influence on culture: relationship with self, relationships with team members, and relationships with patients and families.

- The eight dimensions of the RBC framework are healing culture, patients and families in the center, leadership, teamwork, interprofessional practice, care delivery, system design, and evidence. This book is organized according to these eight dimensions.

- The current language of your organization's cultural narrative reveals a great deal about your culture. Taking care to use language that promotes healthy cultural practices will help advance the culture.

SECTION ONE
Healing Cultures and
Patients and Families in the Center

The most basic and powerful way to connect to another person is to listen. Just listen.

RACHEL NAOMI REMEN

Chapter One

A Relationship-Based Way of Being

Michael Trout and Mary Koloroutis

Who is the most relationally proficient person you know? You may not have heard the term *relationally proficient* before, but we're confident you understand the question. Who do you know who makes a practice of really tuning in to people? Who do you know who is genuinely curious about people? Who is adept at focusing on what a person says and asking questions that help that person get to the core of an issue? Who do you know who feels, to you and others, like a living, breathing safe haven?

Nearly everyone demonstrates a high level of relational proficiency at least some of the time. There are people with whom nearly all of us just find it easy to connect. The difference is that for the truly relationally proficient, there's nothing conditional about the willingness to connect; it's not dependent on how much we like the other person. Being relationally proficient becomes part of who we are. While it may be true that a few of us are born with such capacity or are nurtured in our families of origin such that relational proficiency is second nature to us, it is also true that it can be learned.

Take a look at the practices mentioned in that first paragraph: tuning in, being curious, engaging with what the person says, being a safe haven. These are relational practices, and they are learnable skills.

But are these practices necessary components of exceptional care? We have come to understand that they are necessary if care is even to be called adequate.

While these relational practices are more than mere tools, they are *in fact* tools, and when used properly, they're tools that make some very important things happen. If we use the tool of tuning in—or *attuning*—to someone, the person feels seen because she *is* seen. She feels as though she matters, and, interestingly, the more attuned attention you pay to the person, the more you will come to care about the person (Goleman, 2013). If you use the tool of genuine curiosity—if you *wonder* with and about a person—the person feels as though he is worthy of your interest, and, again, he feels as though he matters to you. If you use the tool of hooking in, with genuine interest, to what the person says or does—the tool called *following*—the person experiences that you are not only working for him but that you are working with him to find a solution or to get him some relief. If you use the tool of creating a safe haven—the tool of mentally and emotionally (and sometimes physically) *holding* the person—the person will feel safe with you (Koloroutis & Trout, 2012).

The more attuned attention you pay to the person, the more you will come to care about the person.

The practices that create and nurture relationships with patients and families are attuning, wondering, following, and holding. As we teach these practices, we have noticed that there seem to be few if any people who have adopted the therapeutic practices of attuning, wondering, following, and holding in their work with patients and families who have not also embraced them in their relationships with their own families, friends, and co-workers. They are not merely "therapeutic practices;" they're the four practices that create, nurture, deepen, and improve all relationships.

The Four Practices: Attuning, Wondering, Following, and Holding

Attuning

Attuning is the most foundational of all of the practices because without it, the other practices are simply not possible. As you can see from Figure 1.1, presence and attunement create the container within which the other practices occur. Attuning can happen in the absence of the other three practices, but the other three practices cannot happen in the absence of attuning.

Attuning is the action of being present to another; it's often explained as "meeting someone exactly where he or she is." When we are attuned we notice things about the person's way of being. Attuning also helps us notice the impact of our own presence on the other person.

Many of us find "presence" difficult—particularly when we are in environments in which distractions are the norm. What we have discovered in our work, however, is that attuning—the conscious practice of tuning in to someone or even some*thing*— actually facilitates presence. Attuning is a thing you can *do* that helps you to simply *be*.

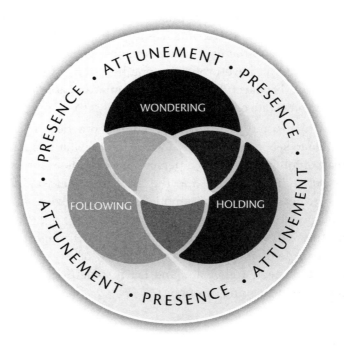

Figure 1.1: The Therapeutic Practices

Wondering

Wondering is a practice of discovery grounded in curiosity and genuine interest in the other. The practice of wondering prevents us from making assumptions, rushing to judgment, or disconnecting from people prematurely. We become more scientific when we wonder. Wondering helps us to resist hasty conclusions, welcome and seek new data, and imagine possible explanations beyond the apparent ones. When we wonder, we miss less and notice more.

When we wonder, we miss less and notice more.

Following

Following is the practice of quiet listening and attending to the rhythm and flow of a person's words as much as to their content. It's what a parent does in the middle of the night when arriving in the room of his crying infant. It's what you have probably done hundreds of times, when you were mysteriously peaceful and aware and quiet and able to truly observe another person's state of mind and body.

Following is usually the hardest relational practice to grasp, but you may be able to see it more clearly by looking at what people sometimes do instead of following. When a person expresses fear, for example, following is *not* saying, "You'll be fine; the doctor is on her way." Following is allowing the person to have his emotions, acknowledging them, perhaps asking for more information, squeezing a hand more tightly, or even just allowing the reality of what the person is going through to register on your face. In order to follow, you have to be able to be with people in their distress, and respect, appreciate, and learn something about who they are and what they're going through.

Holding

Have you ever wondered why nearly every baby on the planet goes through a period in which she says, every day, "Hold me" (often shortened, in baby-speak, to something like "Hold!" or "Up!")? We may worry that it implies too much dependency, or we may think it's just annoying, or we may love it. As the child grows, the daily requests usually go away, but the feeling may not. It may return at any age when one is again vulnerable, and so the need for holding (physically or metaphorically), whether we like it or not, is a key element of relationships. We have the power to help another to reexperience this primal safety net by being a person upon whom he can emotionally rely. We hold someone when we do what we said we'd do. We hold when we remember the things people tell us and perhaps act on them. We hold when we listen without defense or retort.

The purpose of deconstructing these interactions and giving definition to the individual practices that comprise them is to take the mystery out of what constitutes effective relationships. Through the study of these four practices, authentic connection can be learned, reflected upon, practiced, and mastered.

Is This a New Idea?

Consider this illustration: You're standing in an elevator. Two others are with you. They're strangers, but within seconds of their entrance into your space, your nervous systems begin to communicate. You may even be aware that you are taking in data about the fearfulness or sorrow that shows on the face of one of them or about the unusual gait or motor tic of the other. Dozens of other cues are being exchanged too, the vast majority of them at a level below awareness. This capacity is called *neuroception*. Think of it as your brain perceiving something directly, without necessarily engaging your mind. Neuroception is astonishingly effective at helping us ferret out "safety cues" (Porges, 2004). We collect data about one another's heart rate, respiration, affect, even smell. We're looking (again, at a level below awareness) for the state of mind or intention of the other. Depending on our own experiences in life, we attach meaning to these cues: Does this sort of respiratory rate suggest the other is calm, or does it suggest we're about to be attacked?

The elevator stops at the fourth floor. You have two more floors to go. A new person enters. Discernment through neuroception begins anew. We look for, acquire, and analyze a few dozen new bits of physiological and affective data. We start to formulate conclusions. Some of them are wrong; we misperceive a cue, or we attach the wrong meaning to it. But

Seeking to know the other, if only for self-preservation, is something we humans have been doing quite naturally for tens of thousands of years.

we keep at it, and we don't even know we're doing it.

This is really just a story about how natural it is for nearly all of us to perceive the world around us. The study of neurobiology shows us that our capacity for the relational practice of attuning, in particular, is nothing new. It turns out that seeking to know the other, if only for self-preservation, is something we humans have been doing quite naturally for tens of thousands of years. Our neurology appears to be set up in such a way that the leap to a more conscious version of perceiving the world around us—the leap to consciously practicing attuning, wondering, following, and holding—is a very small leap indeed.

The only question on the table is this: Would we prefer to be oblivious to all this neuroceptive activity (Porges, 1995, 1997, 1998, 2001), or would we like to be aware of it—maybe toward the end of using it to improve literally all of our relationships?

What Will the Four Relational Practices Do for You?

Someone is yelling at you. You begin to flare: "How dare he? I don't deserve to be talked to this way! It's not even my fault."

All of your reactions may be valid, no matter what the loud complaint is about; indeed, it's probably *not* your fault. But does establishing the validity of your reactions improve the situation for either of you? You notice that it doesn't.

Enter the tools: attuning, wondering, following, and holding.

You calm yourself and tune in to the person. You get curious rather than making assumptions or judging her. You begin to earnestly wonder. Your heart rate returns to something resembling normal. You get quiet. You find that you're strangely and suddenly adept at following what this person is saying, even though a minute ago, it mostly sounded like loud and challenging words, without actual content. And then, of all the bizarre and irrational things, you find yourself engaging in a momentary act of holding; you breathe deeply and say (or think), "You know what? If I were going through what you're going through, I might feel exactly the same way."

You've gone from flailing to anchored. The relational practices of attuning, wondering, following, and holding have brought you to a quieter state of being. This, we are hearing from those who have studied these practices over time, is the great gift of the relational practices. The practices help you move mindfully from judgment to empathy.

In a care setting, the widespread application of these practices gives people a common language with which to talk about therapeutic relationships. This is the key to making the practices repeatable and refinable. We finally have language that allows people to coach and develop those who have learned, in school and at work, exactly what was taught to them about how to be good clinicians, which may not have included much if any content on how to establish and nurture therapeutic relationships.

The application of these practices isn't, however, limited to improving clinician-patient relationships in care settings. Remember that a few pages ago you were introduced to the three key relationships in Relationship-Based Care: relationship with self, relationship with team, and relationship with patient and family. The four relational practices are just as valuable when applied to one's relationships with self and team as they are in one's relationships with patients and families.

The four relational practices are just as valuable when applied to one's relationships with self and team as they are in one's relationships with patients and families.

Applying the practices in one's relationship with self will be addressed in depth in Chapters Two and Three, where the practice of self-attunement is particularly emphasized. Plato's admonition to "know thyself" is widely accepted as a fine idea, but it's not exactly a how-to. Attuning, wondering, following, and holding, in one's relationship with self, are the how-to. Self-knowing (or self-attunement) enables you to understand your own responses to the people and circumstances around you. It is next to impossible to maintain a sense of composure in challenging circumstances without self-attunement.

The benefits of applying the four relational practices in teams are discussed in depth in Chapter Nine, but they boil down to this: The reason to apply the four relational practices in teams is that they make every interaction smoother and more effective. Because attuning, wondering, following, and holding improve all relationships, they have the power to improve team functioning in ways that are hard to calculate. If even one person in a relationship is attuning, wondering, following, and holding, the relationship will be improved. If two or more are adept at the practices (or are even attempting them), the impact can be transformative.

As people begin to practice attuning, wondering, following, and holding in a health care setting, the language of the practices enters the cultural narrative of the organization, department, or work area. People start talking about how they didn't get triggered by someone's anger because they "*wondered* rather than moving right into judgment" and realized there was a backstory in play, even if they might never come to know the details of that story. People start talking about how they *followed* just a little bit longer than usual: "Normally, I'd have started reviewing the rules and consequences for absenteeism with him right away, but I could see that something was up, so I just stayed present and tried to create a safe haven for discussion. That's when he told me his father with Alzheimer's moved in with his family a week ago . . . and that his wife moved out two days later." There's nothing inherently wrong with leaping right into "reviewing rules and consequences" with people, but it's pretty easy to see how the use of attuning, wondering, following, and holding cannot help but improve every encounter, every time.

Adopting these practices will change the way you think. They'll make you more receptive. They'll help you feel more anchored. They may even make you more courageous. One of our colleagues, a woman who had been practicing attuning, wondering, following, and holding for more than five years at the time of this book's publication, reported:

> The before-and-after is pretty striking for me. I find that "difficult conversations" are no longer difficult for me. My fear had always been that in broaching a tough topic, I might accidentally hurt someone's feelings. That was a big barrier for me, but I don't feel that way anymore. I don't even have to know what I'm going to say. I can just invite someone into a conversation where our only intention is to

wonder together and see what we discover—I often verbalize this as a mutual intention before we begin. It's completely nonthreatening for both of us, and even if the other person isn't aware of the practices, the tension is released. Then I can attune, wonder, follow, and hold my way through anything that comes up.

This same colleague noted also that she now no longer finds herself feeling like she has to persuade people of anything. Before she was skilled at the four practices, when she had a point she felt adamant about, she was afraid of being strident (or being perceived as such); now she finds that it's impossible to be strident when she's attuning, wondering, following, and holding. Not surprisingly, she readily confirmed that all of her relationships have improved significantly since she has become more relationally adept. How could it be otherwise?

It's interesting to us that the use of attuning, wondering, following, and holding in all relationships also seems to foster personal authenticity in people. It's true that you could attempt to use the practices as "techniques," but it is our observation that they don't stay techniques for long. Just as it was, perhaps, only a technique for physicians to "pull up a stool and sit at the bedside at eye level" for a certain number of minutes (Bush, 2011), it was a technique that fostered more authentic connection. It was not that patients and families liked this practice because their doctors sat for a certain number of minutes; they liked it because their doctors connected. Attuning, wondering, following, and holding work the same way. Your motive in adopting these relational practices doesn't matter one bit. If you do them, you will be more authentic in your relationships, and your relationships will improve.

Summary of Key Thoughts

- The practices that create and nurture relationships with patients and families are attuning, wondering, following, and holding. They are not only "therapeutic practices"; they're the four practices that create, nurture, deepen, and improve *all* relationships.

- The relational practices of attuning, wondering, following, and holding can be learned.

- Attuning is foundational to all relatedness. Without it, the other practices are not possible. Attuning is the action of being present to another; it's often explained as "meeting someone exactly where he or she is."

- Wondering is a practice of discovery grounded in curiosity and genuine interest in the other.

- Following is the practice of attending and sometimes responding to the rhythm and flow of a person's words as much as to their content.

- The relational practice of holding happens when we do what we said we'd do, when we remember the things people tell us, and when we listen without defense or retort.

- The study of neurobiology shows us that our capacity for the relational practice of attuning is nothing new. Seeking to know the other—if only for self-preservation—is something we humans have been doing quite naturally for tens of thousands of years.

Reflection

- What are some ways in which you would expect your relationships to change if you were to attune, wonder, follow, and hold more often?

- What might change as the language of the four relational practices enters the cultural narrative of your organization, department, or work area?

If your compassion does not include yourself,
it is incomplete.

THE BUDDHA

CHAPTER TWO

Attuning, Wondering, Following, and Holding as Self-Care

BRETT LONG AND REBECCA SMITH

It is still too rare that individual caregiver health and wellbeing are recognized as critical to clinical outcomes, patient experience, and overall organization success. This oversight persists even though, as most health care leaders realize, it's the *people* in our organizations who create ultimate value for patients—not the latest piece of technology, the most innovative strategic plan, or the grand staircase in the lobby. Yet many of these caregivers are operating at a personal deficit, not feeling fulfilled in life or work (Bartkus & Davis, 2000; Caldwell, 2011; Boyatzis, Goleman, & McKee, 2002; Kegan & Lahey, 2016).

Health care leaders who are called on to transform an ailing industry must feel just as compelled to help transform the ailing caregivers in our organizations if we are to transform the system itself. Caring about the wellbeing of caregivers also makes good financial sense. Depleted and disconnected caregivers impact results in three very tangible ways. First, caregivers who have lost passion for their work are less likely to truly connect with the patients and families in their care (Ahola & Hakanen, 2014; Shanafelt, 2009). Second, individuals working at a personal deficit are more resistant to change, which translates into slower organization improvement cycles and breeds a "we/they" culture (Kegan & Lahey, 2016). And third, direct caregivers who are depleted are more likely to be distracted and to be involved in clinical errors and oversights (Shanafelt et al., 2010).

Relationship-Based Care (RBC) asks us to consider three key relationships that must be healthy in order for organizational cultures to flourish: (1) relationship with self, (2) relationship with colleagues, and (3) relationship with patients and families. The sequence is deliberate. As leaders, it is tempting to put nearly all of our attention on the desired outcome of exemplary patient care, as opposed to thinking through how fundamental the self-care of everyone in the organization is to that vital outcome.

Attuning, Wondering, Following, and Holding as Keys to Understanding and Improving Our State of Wellbeing

For most of us, understanding our level of wellbeing isn't as objective a pursuit as, say, diagnosing an arm fracture: Fall off ladder. Land on arm. Arm aches. Trip to Urgent Care. X-ray. Arm broken. The condition of one's own wellbeing is harder to see so clearly. While many useful assessment tools exist to help you determine your current wellbeing profile, we'd like to invite you to first apply the tools introduced in the preceding chapter. When Trout and Koloroutis explained the four relational practices of attuning, wondering, following, and holding, they laid out not just the route to healthy relationships with others; they laid out a route to a healthy relationship with self. They provide us with four practices that help us to objectively and gently begin an introspective process to identify our current state of wellbeing.

Attuning

Attuning, as a *therapeutic* practice, means getting into a mental and emotional position that allows us to fully understand a person's state of mind and heart. When our aim is *self*-attunement, we want to tune in to our own state of mind and heart.

Take a few seconds to check in with yourself, with your body. Are you feeling settled, grounded, and fully present as you read the words on this page? Are the breaths you're taking deep and long? Or are you feeling distracted, rushed, maybe overwhelmed with work and life—distracted by your internal narrator telling you that you should be doing something else or that you're not working hard enough, spending enough time with your family, helping your aging parents enough, making enough money, making enough of a difference—that *you* are not enough? You probably feel different each day and even moment to moment, but how do you feel most often? If you're like most people, feeling settled and fully present are fleeting feelings, as rare as they are pleasurable. For many of us, being distracted and succumbing to the voice inside—the one that speaks far too often of inadequacies in ourselves—is our default setting.

Attuning requires slowing down, opening to everything around you, and paying attention to subtlety and nuance. The most important thing is to start to be aware of your pace, to commit to slowing down, and to realize that slowing down is actually more efficient. The good news is that it's not an all-or-nothing proposition; you're not either highly self-attuned or completely disconnected from your mind and emotions. You're always, really, somewhere in the middle. As Dan Harris, *ABC News* anchor and author of *10% Happier*, says about his approach to becoming more present through meditation, "Since I have the attention span of a six-month-old yellow lab, I figured [meditation] was something I could never do" (Harris, 2014, p. xiv). But as his book describes, this super-skeptical, New York–based news anchor found his groove and his advantage by creating more space in his life and just plain slowing down. And as he says, if he can slow down, so can you.

As was established in the previous chapter, attuning is foundational to the other therapeutic practices. You can't wonder, follow, or hold if you aren't attuning to someone first. That goes for your relationship with yourself, too. Unless you're willing to attune to yourself, you will not be able to improve your relationship with yourself.

Unless you're willing to attune to yourself, you will not be able to improve your relationship with yourself.

Wondering

Wondering is characterized by curiosity, openness, acceptance, and genuine interest. As suggested in Chapter One, the greatest gift that comes with wondering is that it keeps you from judging prematurely. We'll go a step further and assert that it's actually impossible to wonder and judge at the same time. Wondering prevents judging.

For most of us, the notion of "self-assessment" is practically synonymous with self-judgment or self-criticism. But what would happen if, in your relationship with yourself, you decided that you would simply wonder, with no agenda other than to discover something—*anything*—about the state of your mind, body, and/or spirit?

The relational practice of wondering is a lifesaver for clinicians in therapeutic relationships; think of how much better things go when you move into a sense of wonder instead of judgment in the face of patient or family anger. Think about how good it feels when you're reflecting on a difficult encounter with a colleague, to stay in a state of wonder long enough for some new and soothing insight to make its way into your thought process. When you cultivate the practice of wondering long enough for it to become a habit of mind, it cannot help but increase your compassion for others, and it cannot help but reduce your stress. Now, imagine what it would be like to have a more compassionate relationship with yourself. Perhaps your current self-dialogue sometimes sounds like this: "Ugh! I hate when I do that! What's wrong with me?" Perhaps you will find it less stressful and more productive to think, "Wow, I did _____ again? I wonder what that's all about." You might even want to cap off your gentle inquiry with the always helpful, "I wonder what I'm supposed to learn from this . . . ."

When you cultivate the practice of wondering long enough for it to become a habit of mind, it cannot help but increase your compassion for others, and it cannot help but reduce your stress. Now, imagine what it would be like to have a more compassionate relationship with yourself.

Following

Following can be a little tricky at first. The practice of following requires you to attune, and it helps if you wonder too. (You'll find that the four relational practices overlap a lot of the time.) If you're looking at someone and you're tuned in and curious, it may come to you quite naturally to try to find out more about the person or to ask a question about something the person has said or done. Those are acts of following, but following doesn't just mean asking questions. It's also about responding to and validating the state someone else is in; sometimes it's a concerned look or a loving touch. It is about allowing the other person's agenda to unfold without interruption, without changing the subject, and without rushing to fix the situation. Fundamentally, it is about staying interested and listening.

Now imagine turning that gentle process of inquiry and validation on yourself. Attune to yourself, turn on your sense of wonder, and then follow what you notice. "My shoulders are tense." You rub one of your shoulders, in an act of self-following. You think about how it might have come about that you have tense shoulders. "Maybe too much time at the computer today," you think, in another act of self-following. "This happens now and then, doesn't it? I wonder if there's something specific I've been doing to cause this tension?" Following isn't problem solving; it's not about reaching conclusions. In fact, the practice of following asks you to resist the temptation to automatically place your findings into some sort of story that confirms what you think you already know about yourself. It's simply a practice that allows you to remain open and to pay attention. The practice of following builds relationships—relationships with others or with yourself.

Holding

Holding is, among other things, the natural result of attuning, wondering, and following. In Chapter One, holding someone is equated with creating a safe haven around them. Once you've been working with the four relational practices for a while, you may find that you can create a holding environment for people—a safe haven—simply by consciously intending to do so. (On closer examination, of course, you will discover that you're creating the holding environment by attuning, wondering, and following; you just did them all simultaneously.)

Holding is a wonderful practice to use in your relationship with yourself. Regardless of what you discover about your current state of wellbeing, the practice of holding allows you to accept yourself just as you are. The relational practice of holding, when used on yourself, is an act of self-kindness. It allows you to feel self-respect, self-acceptance, and a sense of dignity, regardless of your state of being.

What Koloroutis and Trout might call self-holding is closely related to what Dr. Kristen Neff calls self-compassion. Neff is a researcher and the author of *Self-Compassion: The Proven Power of Being Kind to Yourself* (2015). Her website greets you with a banner that cuts right to the chase: "With self-compassion, we give ourselves the same kindness and care we'd give to a good friend" (Neff, 2016). Questions such as, "What could I do right now to be more self-compassionate?" are great to have ready whenever you say or think something harsh about yourself. If your aim is to provide a safe haven for others, how much better able will you be to do so if you're working on being a safe haven for yourself at the same time? As we'll see later in this chapter, everything you do, say, or think has an effect elsewhere in the world. If you want the world to feel safe and loving for those in your care, we invite you to start by making your own interior world a safer and more loving place for you.

> *If you want the world to feel safe and loving for those in your care, we invite you to start by making your own interior world a safer and more loving place for you.*

How Attuning, Wondering, Following, and Holding Aid in Healthy Boundary Setting

Some of the benefits of practicing attuning, wondering, following, and holding are obvious: You'll be mindfully present more of the time, you'll find it easier to settle yourself enough to think and act productively (even amid turmoil), and you'll experience a deeper sense of our shared humanity. There is another benefit, however, to which we'd like to give special attention: When you become more adept at attuning, wondering, following, and holding, it will be far easier for you to set healthy boundaries.

As Brett partners with leaders across the country to strategically elevate the role of relationships in the culture, caregivers sometimes share their concern that being continuously open and compassionate isn't sustainable. They feel they must somehow protect themselves from the suffering they observe every day. A physician recently told Brett that she was afraid of "losing herself" if she was too compassionate. The worry about losing oneself in the suffering of others expresses a fear of getting sucked into what seems like a vortex of suffering, never to return. It's not an irrational fear, of course. There is no doubt that the people in our care

are often contending with pain, fear, and grief. The depth of humanity we experience in our work is real.

Still, we have seen people in health care masterfully navigate this challenge. We observe them walking with others in their grief or sadness but not taking it on as their own. While no one group has a corner on what could be called "compassion with boundaries," we do observe that many of those in spiritual care, palliative care, hospice, and oncology are mindful of this continuous challenge and actively working through it. Many of them manage to be openhearted while maintaining good boundaries.

A story from one of our colleagues about a simple interaction illustrates how the relational practices are key to managing an open heart while creating healthy boundaries:

> I was in a grocery store one day when a man, who I guessed to have a traumatic brain injury, approached and started talking to me, amiably, but with intense focus. Situations like this used to make me a little nervous because I didn't know how to balance my desire to give a nice, friendly person some time and attention and my desire to not give nice, friendly people *hours* of my time and attention. Then I remembered attuning, wondering, following, and holding. We spent a few minutes chatting, and the whole time I was cognizant of giving him my undivided attention and zeroing in on what seemed most important to him. I even slowed my breathing in order to really put myself into a space where I could receive him as a person. I committed myself to being undistracted, even though we were in a loud, crowded place. Not a lot of what we said would have made much sense to anyone overhearing us, but we made a nice connection.
>
> After a few minutes, I gently placed a hand near the cuff of his jacket sleeve, kept my eyes warmly fixed on his, and said, "It's been so nice talking with you. I hope we run into each other again." We shared a quiet moment, and then I walked away, keeping a bit of eye contact with him for just a little longer—conveying (I hoped) that our connection wasn't being broken so much as it was being put on hold until we met again. It felt fine ending the interaction because I

knew we'd spent some quality time together. It was lovely, and then it was over.

Obviously, this was a social interaction rather than a clinical encounter, but there is an underlying principle in this story that applies to clinical encounters as well: It's easier to draw boundaries when you know you've made a quality connection. Our colleague knew she'd given the man something valuable, so she felt fine ending their interaction.

Koloroutis and Trout (2012) are very clear that the therapeutic relationship is a one-way proposition: "In the therapeutic relationship the clinician offers care, touch, compassion, presence, and any other act or attitude that would foster healing, and expects nothing in return" (p. 27). While we agree that clinicians should not expect anything in return, they no doubt receive plenty from attuning, wondering, following, and holding. What they get doesn't necessarily come from the patient, however; it's more that attuning, wondering, following, and holding end up being as therapeutic for clinicians as they are for patients and families. In the same way your deep affection for someone has at least as big an effect on you as it does on that person (who may not even be aware of your affection), your own attuning, wondering, following, and holding have at least as big an effect on you as they do on others.

It's easier to draw boundaries when you know you've made a quality connection.

When you attune, wonder, follow, and hold, you end up *involved* with people as opposed to merely tending to their care needs. People sense that you are involved because you *are* involved. You also know that you're making a quality connection, so when it's time to move to the next person, you can pause the face-to-face part of the connection without breaking it. If you've given a person who feels lost and vulnerable the sense that you're in it with him, you've created a safe haven for that person, and that safe haven doesn't disappear when you leave. Because the person feels seen and received, it stays with him.

Perhaps there is some kernel of common sense embedded in the idea that to keep from burning out you'd better keep tight reigns on your compassion, but we invite you to revisit this logic. It's as though you're committing to bringing only your "professional self" to work—not the part of you that houses a full range of human emotions, not your complete self.

While it's true that not every *expression* of every emotion is appropriate at work, it's equally true that your feelings, whatever they are, are valid. It's also very likely, given your work, that you would benefit from spending some time looking closely at your emotions, wondering about them without judgment, and affirming that the reason you sometimes have emotions such as fear, disgust, heartrending compassion, or an almost soul-crushing feeling of inadequacy is that you are a human being working in an environment where tragic things happen every day.

The Fractal Nature of Organizations (or Why Your Level of Self-Care Matters to Everything and Everybody)

If you Google *fractal*, here's what you see:

frac·tal
/ˈfraktəl/ ◀))

MATHEMATICS

noun

1. a curve or geometric figure, each part of which has the same statistical character as the whole. Fractals are useful in modeling structures (such as eroded coastlines or snowflakes) in which similar patterns recur at progressively smaller scales, and in describing partly random or chaotic phenomena such as crystal growth, fluid turbulence, and galaxy formation.

adjective

1. relating to or of the nature of a fractal or fractals.
   "fractal geometry"

︾ Translations, word origin, and more definitions

If fractals are helpful in figuring out how coastlines change, we think they are also helpful in explaining how organizations change. At the risk of oversimplifying this idea, to look at something as a fractal is to realize that every part of a thing is also a representation of the *whole* thing, and every whole thing is also a representation of its parts. For example, if only a small part of a 100-mile coastline changes, the whole coastline is changed. In fact, it could be that only a 10-foot stretch of a coast is radically changed. If you zoomed out and looked at the entire coast, you'd be hard-pressed to notice the difference, but the bottom line is that the shape of the coast is now different, simply because a 10-foot stretch of beach has changed. The corollary is that because you are part of your organization, when you change, your organization changes. It scales up in such a way that a very big change in you can mean a very small, possibly imperceptible change in your organization, but the organization is changed nonetheless.

There are implications to this reality, and some of them are more positive than others. On the negative side, it means that if you believe that your lack of self-care isn't hurting anyone but yourself, you are mistaken. Remember, the entire shape of your organization changes (though perhaps imperceptibly) every time you do. On the positive side, if you bring self-awareness to your organization, your organization is more self-aware. If you bring attunement to your organization, your organization is more attuned. If you bring love to your organization, your organization is more loving.

The Leader's Role in Supporting Individual Self-Care

As physician/philosopher Albert Schweitzer said, "Example is not the main thing in influencing others, it is the only thing." More than any other individuals, an organization's leaders set the tone of its culture. They have the eyes and ears of the organization on them more often than anyone else does, and their example is followed by many in the organization, whether they realize it or not. If leaders are working themselves to a frazzle and expecting others to do the same (whether they say so or not), a culture is advanced in which *the work is more important than the people*. We're talking about cultures in which people are celebrated for working 16 hours straight, answering e-mails at midnight, and not taking vacations. While the leaders of these organizations might be fostering a culture of high productivity and self-sacrifice (which can sound noble if you don't look at it too closely), they're also fostering a culture of self-neglect. If this sounds like the culture you're currently working in, we invite you to pause for a moment to remember, with no small measure of compassion, how well-meaning those who have fostered your current culture almost certainly are. Nobody sets out to create a culture in which people aren't able to take adequate care of themselves or one another. In a world as rushed as health care, such a culture can easily emerge unless the advancement of a culture that includes self-care as a stated and demonstrated value becomes a strategic priority.

The Shadow Every Leader Casts

The workload of health care leaders is immense. We feel confident in stating that the *responsibility* load of every health care leader is even bigger. If our brief foray into fractals taught us that even the least visible person in the organization cannot help but influence the whole organization, it also teaches us that those who are most visible typically have the largest effect on the whole. The ability to influence culture is amplified by positions of leadership. This is a huge responsibility. Highly successful leaders respond to this responsibility as an extraordinary opportunity. If you want to be part of an organization comprising people who are passionate about the shared noble cause of health care, spend time asking people to tell you what they love about their work. If you want to see more people pausing, settling in, and taking a deep breath before they speak, model those behaviors. If you want people in your organization to unfurrow their brows, unfurrow yours.

If you want people in your organization to unfurrow their brows, unfurrow yours.

If you, as a leader, state that self-care is important, then it's important to also model it by visibly putting your own family first and by supporting the colleague who lets you know that he needs to be 20 minutes late for your 8:00 a.m. meeting because he will be dropping his kids off at school. A leader must assert that self-care is a value and then prove it again and again. If you want to work in an organization where people are connecting with their passions, it's up to you to make room for conversations about what people are passionate about. A good leader is not in the business of creating a compliant, obedient workforce. A good leader leads to nurture, in her colleagues, a higher purpose and a commitment to a shared noble cause. A good leader is looking for how the passions of everyone in the organization can contribute to that cause.

None of this is possible unless you bring your whole self to work. None of this is possible while you're holding your breath instead of, at least occasionally, breathing deeply and settling into your physical body.

A Call to Action to Everyone in Health Care

We'd like to offer one final invitation in this chapter: Be your real self at work—your *whole* self.

Who are *we* to issue such a bold and provocative invitation? We're your colleagues, we're your friends, we're your family members, we're your employees, and we're your patients. We've spent enough time with the extraordinary people of health care to know that the real you—the whole you—is who we want taking care of us if we're sick, or designing our organization's care delivery system, or making the financial decisions in the institutions in which we work. We want to interact with your complete self—the one with a full range of human emotions.

We've spent enough time with the extraordinary people of health care to know that the real you—the whole you—is who we want taking care of us if we're sick, or designing our organization's care delivery system, or making the financial decisions in the institutions in which we work.

Because you are a human being working in an environment where tragic things happen every day, more is being asked of you than of people who work in nearly any other setting. If the notion of opening yourself to the full reality of what's happening around you reconnects you with your passion to serve, you're in the right place. Take a deep breath, settle into your skin, and check in with yourself about how you're feeling right now. How do you *really* feel?

Summary of Key Thoughts

- Health care leaders who are called to transform an ailing industry must feel just as compelled to help transform the ailing caregivers in their organizations as they are to transform the system itself.

- Attuning, wondering, following, and holding can all be practiced in our relationships with ourselves.

- When our aim is self-attunement, we want to tune in to our own state of mind and heart. Self-attuning requires slowing down, opening to everything around you, and paying attention to subtlety and nuance.

- It's impossible to wonder and judge at the same time. When you consciously wonder about yourself—particularly when you stay in a state of wondering rather than rushing to conclusions—you keep self-assessment from becoming self-judgment or self-criticism.

- Self-following means checking in with yourself about how you feel physically, emotionally, mentally, and spiritually; validating all of your findings; and staying present to all you discover.

- Self-holding means that you are your own safe haven. It means you have as much compassion for yourself as you have for your most beloved friend or family member.

- When you become adept at attuning, wondering, following, and holding, it becomes easier for you to set healthy boundaries because it's easier to draw boundaries when you know you've made a quality connection.

- Because you are part of your organization, when you change, your organization changes. This means that the more conscious you become, the more conscious your organization (as well as the entire world) becomes.

- A leader must assert that self-care is a value and then prove it again and again. If you want to work in an organization in which people are connecting with their passions, it's up to you to make room for conversations about what people are passionate about.

- Be your real self at work—your *whole* self.

Reflection

- Understanding healthy boundaries is important to our ability to connect with others. Reflect on strategies you use in order to be present and compassionate with others without taking on their emotional state.

- The discussion of fractals reminds us that everything we think, say, or do affects others. This means that everybody matters because together we create the whole. What exactly would you like to see more of in your culture, and what are you willing to do about it?

We don't bless the world out of our expertise. We bless it out of our humanness and shared vulnerability.

RACHEL NAOMI REMEN

CHAPTER THREE

Attunement as the Doorway to Human Connection

MARY KOLOROUTIS AND MICHAEL TROUT

Before All of This

Before I was relegated to endless hours in waiting rooms,
At your mercy for word about my future,
Unable to leave ...

Before I gave you my clothes
And along with them,
My dignity ...

Before my voice got weak ...

Before I lost my full name,
And for some, became my disease ...

Before I lost track of any semblance of rhythm
In my day
And social order in my life ...

Before I meekly gave over my power to people in special clothes
That identified them as experts,
While I fell out of my own uniform
Appearing now, pathetic and of no account ...

Before that,
I was a businessperson with whom people made appointments,
And they took care to be on time with me.

I was a person who took care about how I dressed.
It mattered to me.
Rarely did my rear-end hang out.

I was a person whose voice was strong and respectable.
I never whined.
I didn't need to.
And I didn't much like people who did.

I was a person whose name meant something
In my church,
At my office.

It also meant something to me
To be called by that name,
Although I took it for granted,
Until I lost it.

I was a person who said what he meant,
But would never rage at you.
I knew helplessness and guilt,
But they had never before turned me into someone I no longer recognized.

I was a person with a schedule,
A way of doing things,
A way of being with people.
I could depend on these things.
They mattered to me.

I was a person who was sure of himself.
I didn't usually give away my power,
And I sure didn't give away my underwear.
I wasn't normally lying down when I talked to people,
And I sort of assumed that most folks and I
Shared reasonably equal spots on this planet;
I wasn't above them,
They weren't above me.

Can you imagine me as I was then?
Before I came here
And it all changed?

Can you open your mind
To the idea that
I'm not myself when I'm here?

Can you become curious about who I was?
Who I am,
Despite all of the things I seem to have become here?

Can you see me as a person?

—Michael Trout

The narrator of this poem invites us to enter the world of a patient. It's a world in which a person must give himself over to the care of others. It's a world in which a person worries about the loss of self, a world in which his familiar role as an organized business leader and decision maker becomes a mere background story to his role as patient. The person in this poem invites us to connect with what it feels like to be pulled out of our normal lives and into a situation that changes everything. Perhaps more than anything, it reminds us that what may be routine for caregivers is rarely routine for those receiving care. If caregivers fail to hold that truth front of mind, the person—the human being behind the diagnosis, the trauma, the illness—will feel lost.

Understanding the Non-Ordinary State

Being sick puts a person into a non-ordinary state. Just how non-ordinary depends on things we may overlook in the moment: Are all of his body parts still in place? Can she move? Can he take care of basic bodily functions? Do people still take her seriously? To what extent are his dignity and his sense of competence intact? How dependent does she feel? Who is in charge of his care ... and who is in charge of *him*?

Being in a non-ordinary state heightens a person's need for human connection. When we feel helpless, we may be reminded of how tenuous our grasp is on adulthood. It may terrify us. It may bring on regressive behavior—being prone to anger, for example.

Being in a non-ordinary state heightens a person's need for human connection.

For most of us, it's not difficult to accept vulnerability in children, nor any of the behaviors that arise from it, including crying, raging, making rash decisions, or being discourteous. It may, however, be more of a stretch for us to accept the same behavior in ourselves or in other adults, even when the behavior arises from the same feelings of dependency, fear, extreme vulnerability, or need. An adult who is this vulnerable—this out of tune with his ordinary way of being—looks strange to us. We want to correct the behavior and bark: "Be nice! Stop whining!"

When an adult makes his fear or vulnerability known, we may respond with astonishment, irritability, a loss of creativity about available practical actions, and (let's face it) a reduction in empathy. At a moment when human connection matters most in caregiving, it may be least available to the patient and most elusive to the caregiver. The man lying in the bed in a non-ordinary state, scared to death about his upcoming surgery, ashamed of being so afraid, suddenly feeling as if he has no control over his life or his body, may rage at the nurse who fails to arrive in the room quickly enough. That he needs gentle soothing would be entirely obvious to us if he were a baby, and we would know just what to do. But he's a grownup, isn't he? Why doesn't he just pull himself together?

It's because non-ordinary states make us behave in non-ordinary ways.

If we are able to understand the non-ordinary state of a patient, we become less likely to take personally the patient's non-ordinary behavior. And if we tune out the "noise" in each complaint, we may be able to tune in to what is really going on: She's worried that her insurance won't cover the procedure she needs. He's frightened of needing additional heart surgeries after this one. She doesn't know how she's going to deal with this new diet they're talking about. He is afraid of the pain.

If in the moment we can't fully understand the non-ordinary state of a patient, we can at least listen for a quiet voice from somewhere, that will help us know what is going on in front of us. Paul Kalanithi was a chief resident in neurological surgery at Stanford University when he was diagnosed with lung cancer. He had never smoked, loved the outdoors, and was physically active until unexplained weight loss and severe back pain caused him to see a doctor. CT scan results revealed multiple tumors. Nothing would be the same from that moment on. Kalanithi wrote, "It occurred to me that my relationship with statistics changed as soon as I became one."

Non-ordinary states make us behave in non-ordinary ways.

In his posthumously published memoir, *When Breath Becomes Air*, he spoke of instantaneously traversing the geography from physician to patient. From this new vantage point, he thought about how he interacted with his patients before becoming a patient himself. He practiced medicine full throttle, distracted and disconnected. "I had pushed discharge over patient worries, ignored patients' pain when other demands pressed. The people whose suffering I saw, noted, and neatly packaged into various diagnoses—the significance of which I failed to recognize—all returned, vengeful, angry, and inexorable" (Kalanithi, 2016, p. 85). Now he was living *inside* of suffering, vengefulness, and anger. It was a free-fall, away from the life he imagined and into a life that was foreign and uncertain.

Kalanithi articulated for us the experience of being thrust into a non-ordinary state. It changed everything: destabilizing perspective, emotions, and basic coping mechanisms and creating a whole new set of unwanted physical dependencies. In this non-ordinary state, what Kalanithi sought from health care professionals was not simply scientific knowledge but affirmation that *he the person* mattered—that his life mattered.

Being able to understand that the patient is a person in a non-ordinary state is the first step toward responding with empathy and practical action. We begin to access a therapeutic consciousness. We remember that this non-ordinary state is a normal human response to illness. We recall that it is characterized by anxiety, fear, powerlessness, grief, loss, pain, and difficulty coping. Then we are free to be fully present to someone who is in a non-ordinary state.

The Call for a Non-Ordinary Response

> My mother had just received unexpected news about my father's risk for a procedure and potential prognosis. We were outwardly grieving and displaying emotion. A particular nurse noticed our distress and embraced our grieving group, slowly moving us to a private, quiet room from a very noisy hallway. Her voice was soft and compassionate, and she told us she would check in with frequent updates. She looked so kindly into my mother's eyes and held her hand briefly; she offered us water and told us we could use the room as long as we wanted to. She followed through with her promise, and in that small act of kindness I knew my father was in good hands, and more importantly so did my mom. (Koloroutis, 2017)

For those who are tuned in to the non-ordinary state of patients and their families, the compassionate and loving care rendered by the nurse in this description appears to be an obvious and natural response. Wouldn't any caregiver respond to the grief and distress the nurse witnessed in the same way? Isn't compassionate care the essence of the work of clinical professionals? For many devoted clinicians, the answer is, "Yes, of course." Like the nurse in this story, such clinicians attune by noticing the distress in a grieving group of family members. These clinicians wonder and follow and hold by checking in frequently, using gentle touch, offering water, following through with promises, and safeguarding privacy. Such clinicians see the suffering people before them. The routines of care are simply a backdrop to the *persons* needing care. This nurse and clinicians like her have a practice that is anchored in an ethic of caring (Bergum & Dossetor, 2005; Charon, 2008; Gilligan, 1998; Noddings, 2003).

We have a moral commitment to protect and preserve human dignity and to never reduce a person to the status of object.

An ethic of caring is grounded in the universal truth that we are all part of an interdependent human community. As human beings, we all experience moments of vulnerability and suffering. An ethic of caring is built on the premise that as health care professionals, we have a moral commitment to "protect and preserve human dignity and to never reduce a person to the status of object" (Koloroutis & Thorstenson, 1999). The ethic of caring is integral to professional codes of ethics and is expressed in language that calls for safeguarding human dignity, keeping the focus on the person receiving care, and advocating for the health and safety of those receiving care (American Medical Association [AMA], 2016; American Nurses Association [ANA], 2015; American Occupational Therapy Association [AOTA], 2015). An ethic of caring obligates clinicians to remember that they are never simply treating a physical body.

In relationship-based cultures, compassionate care is developed, actively encouraged, and expected. Leaders model caring interactions and cultivate a community of healers in which all members of the team are seen, supported, and valued for the way their work contributes to human caring. Clinicians are supported to develop and deepen the knowledge, skills, and mindsets that lead to therapeutic connections with those they serve. Awareness of the ethical mandate for humane and compassionate care is cultivated in the work culture through a clearly articulated mission and through ongoing inquiry and reflection.

Bergum and Dossetor, in *Relational Ethics: The Full Meaning of Respect* (2005), propose that a practice of self-questioning is critical to maintaining an ethical awareness. Such self-questioning is straightforward but not easy. It calls for a willingness to question ourselves about what it means to be human and vulnerable. How should we treat each other? Are we caring for the whole person? What do we need to notice that we may not be seeing? What is this person's family asking for? What is important about this person's past experience? Am I listening and really hearing? What biases are getting in my way? Should I sit a little longer with this worried person? Do I need to listen for a while longer, or do I need to move the conversation in a different direction? Such important questioning, whether with fellow clinicians or as an internal thought process, guides ethical practice and helps develop greater therapeutic consciousness.

The Casual Diminishment of Human Beings

The emergency room was so busy that we spent 7–8 hours being treated in the corner of a hallway, as no examining rooms were available.

The nurse designated as my father's nurse for care and communication was unavailable most of the time, requiring other nurses to sub for her. We later found out that the decision to admit my father for observation was made 2½ hours before it was executed. That meant we remained longer in the high-stimulation emergency room environment (high noise level, bright lights, cold temperature) when we could have been in a quiet warm room with designated staff available and a much more restful environment. We were in the emergency room for 7–8 hours, and my father wasn't asked about his general comfort level. Pillows and blankets were not offered. My father was not asked whether he was hungry or thirsty. (Koloroutis, 2017)

This narrative is a portrait of casual diminishment. *Casual* refers to something that happens or is done by chance, without prior thought or planning—unintentional, unconscious, automatic, routine. *Diminishment* is the act of making a person or thing seem little or unimportant—an objectification of the other person as irrelevant. Not only were this patient and family not in the center of the team's care; their experience was one of feeling invisible. Made to stay in the hallway, they were literally on the margins of care. This scenario is not unfamiliar to us. It can happen in any busy health care setting. It does, however, raise ethical questions: Does this experience represent health care harm? Is it ever justified? Is it preventable? Who is accountable?

Sociologist Daniel Chambliss described the organizational forces that contribute to the diminishment of human beings in health care cultures in his book *Beyond Caring: Hospitals, Nurses and the Social Organization of Ethics* (1996). His research indicates that while it is true that individual clinicians in all disciplines can make choices every day to provide person-centered, humane, and compassionate care, it becomes exceedingly difficult when the organization's cultural norms and functional requirements are not designed to support person-centered care and are in fact designed in such a way that they inadvertently inhibit it. No one intends to see a patient or any person as little or unimportant, but in his study, Chambliss and his team observed patterns of habits and practice norms that casually diminish not only those receiving care but those providing care as well. They described cultural characteristics including routinization, high value on speed and productivity, team incivility, primary focus on technology, and objectifying people as a way of coping with the frenetic pace of health care.

It's impossible to consider Chambliss's findings without feeling empathy or even sorrow for both the caregivers and the patients consumed in such cultures, but it's also not hard to see how these things become cultural norms. Wouldn't it follow that patterns of casual diminishment are, by definition, so subtle that we're not likely to notice them? Pulitzer Prize-winning author Eudora Welty offers a metaphor that could explain why this would happen: "My wish, indeed my continuing passion [is] . . . to part a curtain, that invisible shadow that falls between people, the veil of indifference to each other's presence, each other's wonder, each other's human plight" (1996, p. 11). It's interesting to note that a veil is something we can see through, yet we can also see that it's there. The more we look through it, however, the less we see the veil itself. When we are busy and pressures are high, we are not likely to realize that our vision is being affected by a "veil of indifference," and that's largely because we're never completely or even mostly indifferent. It's more likely that we've momentarily lost just a bit of what it takes to look with eyes wide open at a human being's plight and to remain connected even when immediate resolution is not in our control. It could also mean that we are working within a culture that has grown more callous over time, perhaps because the problems keep coming and the resolutions are few. It could mean that we are working in a culture in which it is deemed acceptable to walk past people who are anxious and suffering, simply because resolution is beyond reach; there is a feeling of helplessness, and so the choice is made to not see.

We bring this forward to point out the ethical obligation of every person working in health care in any capacity to lift the veil of indifference as often and as thoroughly as possible. The veil is lifted through our forthright dialogue and unsanitized reflection. The veil is lifted as we make a conscious effort to connect with our common humanity as individuals, as teams, and as organizations. Without the conscious effort to connect with our common humanity, we'll be driven by the momentum of our

It is the ethical obligation of every person working in health care in any capacity to lift the veil of indifference as often and as thoroughly as possible.

routinized processes rather than being connected with the humanity of the people involved.

Obviously a certain amount of routinization is required and even helpful in health care. Our muscle memory will guide us to reach in the same way each time for a device that we will eventually read in the same way as well. But somewhere in the middle of that action, there is a human being. This fact alone—the presence of a human being (who is, more often than not, in a non-ordinary state)—means that the application of the device must not be routine. In the middle of that largely routine action, we use the device within a unique context created not only by the person in our care but by the relationship we have with that person. This is always the case whether we're conscious of it or not, and it is in fact our consciousness that determines the therapeutic quality of that interaction. If you provide direct patient care, do you bring a therapeutic conscious-ness to taking someone's temperature or blood pressure? If you work in the admitting department, do you bring a therapeutic consciousness to helping someone schedule an appointment or feel better oriented to what's going to happen next? When we remember our shared humanity, our seeing becomes sharper. We remember how powerful connection is for all of us.

We are not suggesting that every routine interaction causes harm. We are, however, suggesting that every routine interaction has the poten-tial to cause harm. And further, we are suggesting that cumulative routine interactions result in more systemic misattunement, and therefore the diminishment of all of the people involved. In the story of the father and daughter who were overlooked in the ER for nearly 8 hours, it is reason-able to assume that many of the clinicians who passed them again and again in the hallway also felt a sense of helplessness and frustration. They wanted the patient to be able to move to the next setting, but they could do nothing about it. There is a detachment that comes from feeling help-less. We believe that when a critical mass of people within an organization reach a certain level of detachment, the system itself becomes misat-tuned. There is a sort of "cultural creep" that happens when one person looks away from someone's suffer-ing, and then another does, and then another. Many organizational cul-tures are created deliberately and

Attunement is the only tool that dependably prevents care from being routine.

are carefully tended; more organizational cultures are created, at least in part, by accident, through sins of omission committed in an atmosphere of well-meaning, fast-moving neglect. Over time, this may become a culture in which avoiding eye contact with people whose problems you aren't in a position to solve is acceptable, and taking extra time to solve problems that aren't part of your workload may get you marginalized.

There are a few things individuals can do in this sort of setting: We believe that the most effective way to mitigate the potential harm caused by routine actions is to consciously and consistently attune to patients and families. If an interaction is perceived as routine by the caregiver, it will be experienced as impersonal by the patient and family because it *is* impersonal. A clinician's conscious attunement prevents any interaction between a patient and clinician from being impersonal. When we are attuned, we are paying attention to the other.

Attunement Is the Doorway to Human Connection

We'd like to propose something rather provocative that we hope you will carry with you as you continue reading this book: Because of the fast pace and the need for some degree of routinization in every health care environment, systemic misattunement will be the default of every institution unless the people within that institution become "students of attunement." Attunement is the only tool that can dependably prevent care from seeming routine to patients and families because it is the only tool that prevents care from *being* routine. This has obvious implications in one-to-one relationships, of course, but we propose that the implications it has across whole organizational cultures are equally significant, though less visible unless consciously sought out.

We realize that the term *systemic misattunement* may be new to you. To better understand it, imagine a clinician who is not very tuned in to the people she serves. Imagine a team that functions without adequate communication and without accountability to one another. Imagine an organization in which systems and processes are designed for the efficient processing of large numbers of patients and in which clinicians are treated as interchangeable parts. You now have a portrait of systemic misattunement. If even one of these factors is in play, patients may experience the whole system as misattuned.

Now imagine a clinician who is highly attuned to the people he serves. Imagine a team of clinicians who communicate well and are highly accountable to one another. Imagine an organization in which processes and structures are designed to maximize the patient's experience of feeling held in the care of a cohesive team. See a system in which attuned relationships are built, coordination of care is clear and effective, and patients have an active say in decision making. This means that the patient will be treated like a person who matters and is central to the provision of care. This is a portrait of an attuned system. Quality and patient satisfaction literature document that the difference in a patient's experience of care in a misattuned system versus an attuned system shows up in patient experience scores. Even more importantly, it can mean the difference between a patient who gets better and a patient who does not (Berwick, Nolan, & Whittington, 2008; Dempsey, 2014; Reid et al., 2010; Riess, 2015).

Attuning to another person means moving into a physical, mental, and emotional position to be able to catch on to a person's state of mind and heart. To attune to someone means to connect with empathy. In a clinical setting, attuning suggests a level of connection (even if temporary) that opens the door for the patient to resonate with the clinician and the clinician to resonate with the patient. In short, therapeutic connection does not happen without attunement.

Now let's take what we know about attunement and apply it to the portrait of systemic misattunement in the story of the father and daughter in the ER. If we agree that it is never acceptable to leave people on the margins, then we must apply this tool of attunement in a more systemic way. For example, when the ER gets backlogged, and we can't send people on to a unit, the question becomes what *can* we do? This is an important question that calls for a proactive design. For example, we may design a "code compassion" in which a backup team is called to be emotionally and practically supportive to the patient and family, and, by extension, to the care team (Koloroutis & Trout, 2012, p. 278). This team could include house supervisors, administrators, people from pastoral care and social services, and others whose job it would be to connect with the people affected and listen to them, communicate updates, and provide them with basic comfort items such as extra blankets and water. This wouldn't be a problem-solving team per se; if there are no beds, there are no beds. This would be an attunement team, designed to assure patients that they have not been lost in the shuffle. In the same survey from which both of the patient stories in this chapter were harvested (Koloroutis, 2017), we found consistent evidence of how little it takes for patients to feel seen and held. A designated team that went into action for a code compassion would solve the number one problem of patients and family members who are feeling lost and overlooked: the need for human connection.

Interestingly, the establishment of a code compassion would solve the number one problem of the caregivers in this scenario as well: the need to feel as though they're making a positive difference. No clinician thrives when she feels as though the safest course of action is to keep her head down and avoid eye contact so as not to get drawn into trying to solve a problem that's beyond her control. When we cope by shutting people out, the pain is exacerbated for everybody. Imagine how the father and daughter in our story would have felt if they'd been approached by a concerned person a few times over the course of their long stay. Imagine also how the care team's experience would have improved. In both cases, it's a sense of isolation that increased their suffering; compassionate connection with clear communication could have done much to alleviate suffering for all concerned.

No clinician thrives when she feels as though the safest course of action is to keep her head down and avoid eye contact so as not to get drawn into trying to solve a problem that's beyond her control.

Attunement Leads to Better Quality and Safety

The gifts of attunement to clinicians, patients, and patients' families are innumerable. Attunement is a feeling of harmony or oneness with another being; it is both a way of being and a way of doing. It's the experience of focusing on another person with openness and acceptance (Koloroutis & Trout, 2012). When you are attuned to your patient, the patient experiences that you are truly present, and she feels emotionally safe. Attunement also results in better quality and safer outcomes.

Attunement is the doorway to having a therapeutic connection with the person, which leads to better quality by improving the accuracy of assessment, diagnosis, treatment, and overall efficacy (Doyle, Lennox, & Bell, 2013; Lown, Rosen, & Marttila, 2011; Riess, 2015).

There are some guiding principles for safer, higher-quality care that all clinicians know but that sometimes fall by the wayside in fast-paced care environments. For one, our chances of getting the diagnosis and ongoing assessment right are much improved when we know the patient. A disease (a syndrome, a condition, an illness, a problem) never exists outside the context of the person. In order to gain access to the person, we must be willing to engage with that person. When we do not engage—when, for example, attunement to the whole person is not a priority during diagnosis and ongoing assessment—we are prone to make mistakes in diagnosis and ongoing assessment. In other words, if we don't really look, we don't really see.

If we don't really look, we don't really see.

No wise clinician would recommend a course of treatment for a middle-aged woman complaining of headache (or worsening of her arthritis, or depression, or weight gain or loss) without asking the obvious questions about duration, including wondering about when, if ever, these symptoms have appeared before. This is not a routine, innocuous line of questioning. We are really saying, "These symptoms are happening to a *person*. I want to know that person because I can't help unless I do." So we ask her about it in earnest, and we ask as if the human connection we establish when we earnestly ask is as important as anything else we will do this day with this patient. Often, answers come, but even when they don't, a connection is created between patient and clinician when they jointly set out to discover what's wrong. The clinician becomes someone dependable. The patient becomes someone of interest, someone memorable.

Another guiding principle we'd like to lift up is that the patient is safer if we make the human connection that is necessary to understand what is going on with the whole person. We all claim adherence to standards of safety in health care, but have we acknowledged that safety is dependent on a number of factors that are somewhat out of our control unless we take specific actions? If the patient does not fully disclose information about his condition, behavior, symptom changes, or adherence to the recommended protocol—which is easy for him to omit if we're not fully engaged and difficult for him to omit if we are engaged—then we have failed to take the actions needed to protect patient safety. Blaming the patient at that point is a little silly. It is our failure. We did not connect. We didn't look up. We didn't listen and inquire fully. As a result, the patient is less safe in our care.

In a review of evidence from 55 studies, Doyle et al. (2013) conclude that the link between patient safety and highly attuned clinicians is very strong. In a survey of patient experiences with hospital safety, there were fewer medical errors by hospital staff in instances in which patients independently reported that they felt listened to and respected by physicians and nurses in those hospitals ("How Not to Get Sick(er) in the Hospital," 2015, p. 32). We, in turn, conclude that "feeling listened to and respected by physicians and nurses" is the direct result of caregiver empathy, curiosity, scientific persistence, and ultimately, attunement. Likewise, the outcome measures are shifting from a primary emphasis on quality and safety scores to a new, integrated emphasis on quality, safety, satisfaction, and cost of care.

When there is a therapeutic connection between patient and caregiver, patient confidence in the caregiver rises, anxiety declines, adherence to medical guidance increases, and the patient feels seen, heard, and known. He joins with the caregivers instead of resisting them. All of these factors contribute measurably to patient safety, both in the caregiving facility and beyond (Doyle et al., 2013).

Finally, we'd like to remind you that the efficacy of care increases when care is delivered with empathy, in a context of mutual trust. It's surprising how effective empathy is as part of a health care intervention. Patients with new onset of the common cold who had independently rated their caregiver as empathetic (using a protocol known as the Consultation and Relational Empathy scale) experienced reduced severity and duration of their colds, based on IL-8 and neutrophil count (Rakel et al., 2011). Outcome research on 21,000 patients with type 1 or type 2 diabetes showed that those whose physicians received high ratings for empathy (on the Jefferson Scale of Empathy) had fewer acute metabolic complications such as hyperosmolar state, diabetic ketoacidosis, and coma (Del Canale et al., 2012).

In plain language, health care works better in an atmosphere of shared trust, shared purpose, and mutual respect. It's difficult to imagine that we must say this out loud, much less that we must make a case for it. Yet we continue to hear the perspective that our relationship with the patient is somehow separate from (and far less than equal to) the medical care of the patient. There is a lingering perspective that views attunement and empathy as attributes of mere niceness instead of core requirements for the patient getting better, for the department or clinic running better, and for increased efficacy of the entire health care system.

The Million Dollar Question

Since attunement improves clinical quality, is attunement an ethical imperative?

We have said that the therapeutic practice of attunement is the doorway to human connection. We have stated that attunement is a tool and that, just like any other tool, every clinician and person in health care with direct patient contact can learn to use it. This means that human connection in health care (a.k.a. a therapeutic connection), which is achieved through the application of the tool of attunement, is not dependent on the personality traits of the provider. Instead, attunement is a teachable skill that promotes personal and professional meaning and patient wellbeing (Koloroutis & Trout, 2012; Kopp, 2013).

Attunement is a teachable skill.

If all of this is true, do we dare fail to take advantage of this tool? Knowing what is needed for optimal health care, and failing to do it, raises questions of ethics.

Here are some questions for reflection about the use of therapeutic connection as a tool for healing:

- There is evidence that human connection improves health outcomes. Is it, then, an ethical issue if we do not use it?

- When practitioners take it upon themselves to opt out of creating therapeutic relationships because they've decided it's not a good fit for them, is this an ethical problem?

- If we sometimes fail to connect because we conclude we haven't got the time or the energy, even when the evidence is clear that such a failure will actually cause the frustrated and lost patient to use *more* of our time and energy, is that an ethical issue?

First-line caregivers know more about this quiet issue than almost anyone else: that people actually get better and stay better and look after themselves better when someone connects with them. What an astounding capacity for healing lies in the hands, the eyes, the voice of every attuned caregiver.

> *What an astounding capacity for healing lies in the hands, the eyes, the voice of every attuned caregiver.*

Surely we should make the therapeutic application of attunement a priority—first as individuals, then as teams, and ultimately as organizations. Our technical expertise is a great gift, both to us and to our patients. Our relational expertise—our ability and determination to attune to another—is equally a gift, both to our patients and to ourselves.

Connection with Self

We invite you to consider one more ethical question: Dare we commit to human connection as a priority in our provision of health care, while denying the same connection to ourselves? If we determine that it is in fact an ethical imperative that we commit to attuning to others in the provision of health care, is it ethical (or even possible, for that matter) to provide that connection with others if we are not also self-attuned?

One particularly lovely definition of ethics is offered by Kylea Taylor, author of *The Ethics of Caring,* who asserts, "Ethical behavior is reverence for life demonstrated by right relationship to another" (1995, p. 10). But what if we said it this way: "Ethical behavior includes reverence for *our own* lives, demonstrated by right relationship to ourselves"? It's not going to work if you commit to being devoted to your patients while neglecting your own beautiful, suffering heart.

Ethical Actions Create Ethical Environments

A basic tenet of Relationship-Based Care is that the responsibility to create ethical environments belongs to every clinician, administrator, and service person in every health care organization. Ethical environments are fostered by the dignified, respectful interactions, no matter how small, that happen in every corner of the organization. Treating someone with dignity and respect means treating the person like you would want your most precious loved one to be treated. We hear stories all the time about people putting their therapeutic consciousness into action to beautiful effect:

A student nurse cleans the body of a man who has recently died. He speaks to the man gently, despite the fact that the man will never hear anything again, telling him what he is about to do as he cleans his body. All the while he endures, with quiet dignity, the teasing of his nursing assistant partner who thinks he is foolish for speaking to a dead body.

A physician takes the time to ask each patient, every time, "What's most important to you right now?" Then she listens to each answer and asks more questions until she truly understands.

A member of the transport staff at a Veterans Administration hospital finds the room of a newly deceased veteran in disarray, including an American flag strewn carelessly over a chair. He straightens the room and sees to it that the man's body is neatly draped with the flag as he wheels him slowly, ceremonially down the hallway. The man's dignity creates a field in which all who see him stop, make room for them to pass, and salute the veteran until he is out of view. In the weeks that follow, the man works with his unit practice council to establish these actions as standard protocol.

It comes down to a simple but powerful fact: The diminishment of one is the diminishment of all; therefore, each time we act to preserve the dignity of another human being, we preserve our own dignity as well. This is not merely a lovely sentiment. It's how things work in a world where everything is interconnected, where no action exists in a vacuum, where everything is affected by everything else.

Clearly, in order to safeguard the dignity of another, we need to be aware of and attuned to our own human dignity. We need to have a basic understanding of what it means to embody human dignity. It means understanding that in order to embody and preserve dignity in ourselves, we must never trivialize it or permit our organization's culture to allow acts or attitudes to diminish human dignity and respect.

Each time we act to preserve the dignity of another human being, we preserve our own dignity as well.

This generation of health care professionals has an immense opportunity. How wonderful it would be if people could one day say of this current generation, "They were the generation who figured out how to see people as people and to provide humane, compassionate care, even while working in institutions designed to provide services to large numbers of individuals as efficiently and cost-effectively as possible." If we put our hearts, minds, and hands to the work of creating structures and processes that preserve and promote human connection, it may be said of us that we revolutionized health care so quietly and persistently that no one even realized a revolution was taking place.

Summary of Key Thoughts

- Being sick puts a person into a non-ordinary state characterized by anxiety, fear, powerlessness, grief, loss, pain, and difficulty coping.

- Understanding that the patient is a person in a non-ordinary state is the first step toward responding with empathy and practical action.

- Taking on the therapeutic consciousness necessary to be fully present to someone who is in a non-ordinary state is the foundation of ethical health care.

- The process of human relationship is guided by questioning ourselves and one another and by engaging in conversations about what it means to be human and vulnerable.

- Casual diminishment of patients is more likely to occur where we find routinization and focus on tasks instead of focus on the person, high value on speed and productivity, team incivility, a primary focus on technology, and objectifying people as a way of coping with chaos.

- Because of the fast pace and the need for some degree of routinization in every health care environment, systemic misattunement will be the default of every institution unless the people within that institution become "students of attunement."

- Attunement is the only tool that can dependably prevent care from seeming routine to patients and families because it is the only tool that prevents care from *being* routine.

- A disease (a syndrome, a condition, an illness, a problem) never exists outside the context of the person.

- Patients are safer if we take time to make the human connection that is necessary to understand what is going on with them.

- The efficacy of care increases when care is delivered with empathy, in a context of mutual trust.

- When there is a therapeutic alliance between patient and caregiver, patient confidence in the caregiver rises, anxiety declines, adherence to medical guidance increases, and the patient feels seen, heard, and known.

- Attunement is a tool, and everyone in health care can learn to use it. The tool of attunement is not dependent on personality traits but is a teachable skill that promotes personal and professional meaning and patient wellbeing.

Reflection

- Consider the term *casual diminishment*. Can you think of anything in your practice that may inadvertently result in the diminishment of another person or of yourself?

- What would it take to create a "code compassion" within your care team? What would be the components of a code compassion in your setting? What circumstances might call for a code compassion in your setting?

- What would someone who embodied human dignity always do? What would she never do?

- Consider this quote: "They were the generation who figured out how to see people as people and to provide humane, compassionate care, even while working in institutions designed to provide services to large numbers of individuals as efficiently and as cost-effectively as possible." In what ways is this already happening?

Every time you help my family, you help me.

MARCUS ENGEL

CHAPTER FOUR

The Voice of the Family

MARY KOLOROUTIS, MARKY MEDEIROS, AND MARY GRIFFIN STROM

The hospice staff was excellent. Very caring, yet very "to the point" with the information relayed to my brother, my father, and me. The staff explained, very scientifically yet still easy for nonmedical people to understand, what was happening to my mother's body and mind. They also explained the dying process and what to expect. My mom proceeded through the stages, almost exactly as they described. Even though this information was very clinical/scientific, it was delivered with compassion. Something that greatly sticks in my mind: All conversations were free flowing. They allowed us to stop if we were uncomfortable, ask questions at any point, and the staff would follow up with my family very often. These conversations often included information on the dying process. None of the conversations seemed to be a scripted "check-list" that the staff was going through, which once completed, would be checked off the "to do list." They worked with us. Not only did it help us get through the dying process with my mother, I realize it made a difference to us as we grieved for her after her death. With the knowledgeable support of the hospice staff, we feel like we did our very best for her at the end. That is a comfort that is hard to describe.

A SON, ON THE PASSING OF HIS MOTHER (KOLOROUTIS, 2017)

The patient and the family are at the center of Relationship-Based Care. (See Figure 4.1.) This clear inclusion of the family as central to the care experience calls for the health care team to intentionally involve the family in the patient's care when appropriate and to provide therapeutic support to the family. The hospice team described in this adult son's experience epitomized what it looks like to involve and care for the family. They created a therapeutic connection with the family that not only helped them cope with the dying process but contributed to their healing after their loved one's death.

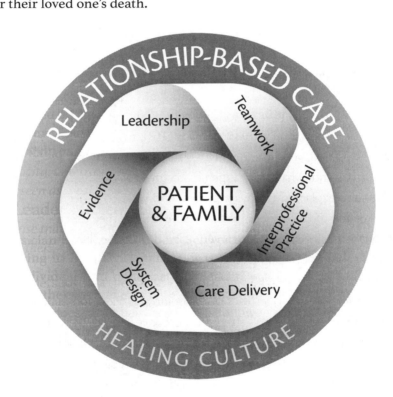

Figure 4.1: Relationship-Based Care Model

When we speak of the family, we speak of anyone the patient determines his family to be. They are the people who are in the patient's life and are affected by the patient's need for care. Family could be the trusted friend who accompanies someone to a clinic appointment. Family could be the friend, sibling, or significant other at the bedside in the hospital—people who find themselves listening closely or voicing concerns on behalf of their loved one. Family members, as identified by the patient, should be welcomed to partner with caregivers to help assure that their loved one is safe and receiving appropriate care.

Research confirms that the presence and participation of family members and friends as partners in care provides cost savings, enhances the patient and family experience of care, improves management of chronic and acute illnesses, enhances continuity of care, and prevents hospital readmissions (Boudreaux, Francis, & Loyacono, 2002; Brumbaugh & Sodomka, 2009; Davidson et al., 2007; Edgman-Levitan, 2003; Fumagalli et al., 2006; Garrouste-Orgeas et al., 2008; Halm, 2005; Lewandowski, 1994; Sodomka, 2006; Titler, 1997).

Family members, as identified by the patient, should be welcomed to partner with caregivers to help assure that their loved one is safe and receiving appropriate care.

The research is also clear that isolating patients at their most vulnerable times from the people who know them best places them at risk for medical error, emotional harm, inconsistencies in care, and costly unnecessary care (Cacioppo & Hawkley, 2003; Clark, Drain, & Malone, 2003). For many older patients, hospitalization for acute or critical illness is associated with reduced cognitive capacity, functional decline, loss of ambulatory ability, and disability related to new activities of daily living at discharge (Ehlenbach et al., 2010; Labella, Merel, & Phelan, 2011). Families and trusted friends are much more keenly aware of any changes in cognitive capacity or functional ability than hospital staff are and therefore are a valuable resource during hospitalization (IPFCC, 2010). The Hospital Elder Life Project (HELP) has identified interventions that can prevent decline, delirium, and falls in hospitalized older patients. A key factor in prevention is the inclusion of the family during the patient's hospitalization and preparation and support of the family caring for their loved one after discharge ("For Family Members," 2016).

Current trends that move clinicians from a philosophy of care that focuses on *doing for* to one that involves *partnering with* have positively impacted the patient experience and improved patient care outcomes (Mastro, Flynn, & Preuster, 2014). Family members of patients are already commonly seen as essential partners in pediatrics, obstetrics, hospice, and home care. It's interesting to note that the clinicians who have led the way in including families as partners are working in settings caring for people at the beginning and at the end of life. But the time has come for care providers to embrace family involvement across the entire spectrum of health care, especially in light of mounting evidence that including the family improves patient safety, patient satisfaction, and patient outcomes.

In this chapter, we offer some insights into what is important to families with loved ones receiving care, as well as ways in which families can be engaged as valuable partners in their loved ones' care. We also hope to ease the perceived "burden" of family inclusion by shifting the mindset from family as additional workload to family as welcome partners in care.

Family Involvement Is Important for Optimal Quality

It's important to remember that the non-ordinary state, as introduced in the previous chapter, extends to the family members of patients as well. One of the barriers to family involvement, admittedly, is clinicians' past experience with the behavior of family members who are distressed and having difficulty coping or who are reacting to a sense of not being heard by those caring for their loved one. In their non-ordinary states, family members tend to be on high alert for danger to their loved ones, and when they perceive, rightly or wrongly, that their loved ones are not getting the help they need, they will do what it takes to "sound the alarm." Sounding the alarm may be the only aspect of care a family member has control over in a system that has a defined set of rules that may or may not appear to meet their needs.

Here is a quote from writer and speaker Marvelyne Engel, wife of author Marcus Engel. Marcus has had hundreds of surgeries over the last two decades following a traumatic car accident that left him blind (Engel, 2010). These are Marvelyne's words:

> I will say that I HAVE been the crazy, frantic lady running down the hallway screaming, grabbing a doctor, literally yanking him into my husband's room saying, "You've got to look at this NOW." In my defense, that was after sitting five hours in the ER, almost two hours in the exam room, not having a doctor in there, and even as a nonprofessional, I knew that a 6-inch incision from a recent surgery

that looked like a football was about to burst through it and had red streaks growing off of it by the moment, was not something that should be happening. It turned out to be a vanco resistant bacteria that had entered my husband's body, and I would run down the hall and be the crazy lady again in a moment, because I HAD to. I was in that position, and I needed to. I hope it never happens again. (Creative Health Care Management, 2013)

Her comments make clear the desperation she felt at seeing her husband's rapid and terrifying decline, and they also make clear that she would do the same thing again if she felt that her husband was in danger. No one wants to be a "crazy, frantic" person, but most of us can identify with doing whatever it takes to protect our loved ones. It is typically only when patients or family members are overcome by feelings of fear and abandonment that they will lose their usual sense of decorum and behave in a way that is far from their ordinary way of being.

It is typically only when patients or family members are overcome by feelings of fear and abandonment that they will lose their usual sense of decorum and behave in a way that is far from their ordinary way of being.

After experiencing a response like Marvelyne's, a care team might be tempted to find fault with this out-of-control family member, but it would be far more productive for the team to get curious. How could this have been prevented? What did we fail to hear? To notice? To communicate? What would have helped the patient and family member feel held? Over time, the inquiry could deepen: What beliefs do the members of the care team have about the role of the family? If family members are not treated as partners, it is clear that they are not *thought* of as partners. And if we're not thinking of family members as partners, how *do* we think of them?

Beliefs about Family Members

While the evidence supporting the value of family involvement is well known in the health care industry and is recognized and promoted as the gold standard of care, the actual experience of involving family members varies widely and, in some health care cultures, is actively resisted. In 2003, a research team from Planetree asked hospital staff to describe the "perfect patient and family." The attributes described were as follows: a passive patient with no family; one who does not ask questions; one who never rings the call bell; one who does exactly what he or she is told; and one who has no visible family members or friends to advocate on his or her behalf (Frampton, Gilpin, & Charmel, 2003). While much has changed since this research, the values and beliefs underlying these responses persist. In some settings, families continue to be viewed as "visitors" (even if the word may be long gone) and as potential obstacles to care rather than a key part of the patient's experience and care.

In an article titled "Using Evidence to Overcome Obstacles to Family Presence," (Davidson et al., 2014) the authors reviewed the evidence surrounding common concerns about family presence. The obstacles to inclusion of the family most frequently cited include "fear of infection and harm to the patient, family interference with the quality of rounds, assumption that families need to go home and rest" (p. 407). The authors took each obstacle listed and used available research to determine whether the obstacle or concern was fact or fiction. Their findings are presented in Figure 4.2.

Concern	Fact or Fiction
Open visiting increases infection.	Fiction
Family presence during procedures increases infection.	Fiction
Family presence in burn patients increases infection.	Fiction
Family presence in the neonatal intensive care unit increases infection.	Fiction
Family presence on rounds is anxiety producing for families.	Partial fact. If rounds are not managed properly, both staff and family may have anxiety. The majority of family members would prefer to be present on rounds.
Family presence on rounds will slow down rounds.	Fiction

Concern	Fact or Fiction
Family presence on rounds will decrease the quality of teaching rounds.	Fiction
Family presence on rounds increases legal risk.	Largely fiction. The risk of confidentiality needs to be managed, but the benefit to the patient and family of improved communication appears worth the risk.
Family presence adversely affects patient physiology.	Fiction
Families should be encouraged to "go home to rest."	Largely fiction. Many families feel the need to safeguard the patient and be present. The need to be present is rated higher by families than permission to go home. If presence is desired, it could be harmful to send them home.

Figure 4.2: Objections to Family Presence: Fact or Fiction? (Used with permission, Davidson et al., p. 418.)

What we know to be true is that any clinician's or care team's firmly held beliefs affect their actions and their interactions. An important first step to any cultural advancement is to assess individual and group beliefs and to challenge the ones that compromise our capacity for connecting therapeutically with those in our care.

James Kelly's compelling book *Where Night Is Day* (2013) is a narrative about life in the ICU. In describing a care conference with a family who was upset that their loved one had not yet been seen by a physician, Kelly writes, "I know Fowler [the attending physician] doesn't believe that no doctor has spoken to them. We think families lie all the time" (p. 20). This author describes a firmly held belief that is prevalent in this unit's culture. If the belief that "we think families lie" is a commonly accepted norm, then interaction with the family would be affected by this belief, which has the potential to shut down curiosity and openhearted attunement. It would make clinicians more likely to look for evidence of untruth and more likely to protect themselves against manipulation by the family. When this happens, important information is less accessible to the clinicians, and the family is less likely to be able to learn what they need to know to care for their loved one.

In a conversation in one of our workshops, an emergency department staff member described a firmly held belief in her care culture that "We need to protect our patients from their intrusive families." This belief aligned with another belief that family presence would interfere with emergency interventions. When asked if this was a perception of families in general or the rare family situation, the response was that this was a belief that colored their perceptions of families in general.

As the discussion unfolded, another clinician offered a very different insight from her own practice:

> First, if we are legitimately concerned that a family member is a threat to the patient's safety, we need to bring that to the attention of the appropriate personnel, to be evaluated by abuse experts. But in most care environments, that is a rare occurrence. In a much more likely scenario, there may indeed be family members who we believe to not be good for the patient, but it is THEIR family, and the patient will return to that family environment, so it seems imperative that we not make judgments about the situation based on our own lives. The patient's family situation is not about us; the onus is upon us as health care providers to provide information, care, and loving attention, alongside and even in partnership with whatever family member the patient deems to be their primary family contact.

Now let's contrast the beliefs of the two workshop participants: For the first clinician, the family is seen as intrusive, and for the second clinician, family members are seen as partners in care, irrespective of their abilities or apparent willingness to partner. The difference between the beliefs that these two clinicians hold is vast, and it takes little imagination to predict how care of the family would differ based on their beliefs. Our beliefs comprise our mindsets, and our mindsets determine our actions, both conscious and unconscious.

Beliefs can be complicated, though, largely because we aren't always fully aware of what we believe. We rarely adopt a belief because of a conscious decision to do so. More often, beliefs build slowly and unconsciously, until one day we find ourselves living our lives differently, for better or worse, from how we lived a decade earlier. Group beliefs build in much the same way. How does it happen that a whole group of clinicians can come to think of families as intrusive rather than as partners in care? It happens, quite reasonably, when people experience what looks to them—and what may actually be—the families of patients creating barriers to patient care. Clinicians are protective, and it may not take many instances of actual family interference to generate the belief that families interfere. The risk is that if these beliefs go unexamined, they harden into biases, and biases shut down curiosity and therefore therapeutic connection. In this particular situation, they keep clinicians from partnering with the patient's family—typically the very people who will take on the responsibility to care for the patient after discharge.

In a debrief of beliefs such as "Families are intrusive," or "That family didn't seem to care," an individual or group could ask, "What would have happened if we'd offered our undivided attention to the 'difficult' family member?" or "What kind of backstory might have been in play with this family?" or "Is it possible that if any one of us had spent a few minutes listening to them, we would have saved everyone a lot of time and trouble in the long run?"

Here's some additional wisdom from the clinician who shared her experience on how and why she makes it a point to involve family members, even if they don't seem to fit the mold of the concerned family caregiver:

> *Better care comes through connection, not isolation.*

> It's on us to stay curious. For all we know, the "difficult" or "apathetic" family member may be triggered mostly by the fact that he feels hopelessly inadequate to the task of taking care of his loved one. Our response, if open, nonjudging, and loving, may be just what this family needs to encourage involvement and participation. Better care comes through connection, not isolation.

What Matters Most to Families

In anticipation of writing this chapter, we surveyed individuals who have had a loved one who recently needed care. We asked them to teach us what mattered most to them in the care of their loved ones with these questions:

1. Which best describes your overall experience with care? (rated "very pleased" to "not at all pleased")

2. Have you experienced moments of anger or frustration with your loved one's care?

3. If you could advise physicians, nurses, or any caregiver to do one or two pivotal things in the care of your loved one and/or in the care team's interactions with you, what would they be? Assume excellent clinical skills are there. Beyond those, what would you like to see caregivers do?

4. Have you experienced moments of deep appreciation for your loved one's care?

We received responses from 53 people. Thirty-seven percent of the respondents identified themselves as clinicians, 35% said they are not associated with health care, and an additional 28% of respondents said they work in health care but are not clinicians. Care was received in settings across the entire continuum: 73% were hospitalized, 11% experienced care in ambulatory settings, 7% in long-term care or rehabilitation settings, 5% in hospice, and 4% in home care. Twenty of our respondents were daughters, 14 were mothers, 11 were spouses or significant others, 4 were sons, 2 were fathers, and 2 were siblings. None of the respondents identified their relationship with the person receiving care as a friendship. What follows are selected responses to the survey questions. They represent a full range of what we learned.

Survey Responses: "Very Pleased with Care"

Forty-five percent of family members report being very pleased with care. Their comments suggest they were very pleased with care when caregivers were present and attuned, when communication was thorough and consistent, and when it was apparent to them that the team was working together on behalf of their loved one. Respondents consistently conveyed that what mattered most to them is that their loved one received compassionate and respectful care and that they were treated with dignity. It was also important to the family that their loved one's comfort and pain needs were addressed quickly. The following comments reflect what is important to them:

- They made a very shy, anxious eight-year-old boy feel like part of the process. The physician's assistant was great at being in the moment and patiently answering our son's questions and concerns.

- Each step of our transition was met with thoughtful, caring team members.

- Everyone in ICU was very kind and thoughtful. They did everything they could to save him.

- I appreciated the way the team told us everything about what was going on; that helped us make our decisions.

- My daughter was in a great deal of pain upon admission. She was triaged quickly, and the nurse immediately began comfort measures. I could see my daughter begin to calm as she knew the nurse believed her and was taking action.

Survey Responses: "Problems with Care" and "Not at All Pleased with Care"

Fifty-five percent of the respondents reported experiencing problems with care; 47% described care as a mixed or marginally satisfying experience; and 8% said they were not at all pleased with care. Reasons for problems included inadequate or unskilled communication, ineffective teamwork, lack of individualized attention, and lack of clinical competence which compromised quality and safety. Here are some of the comments:

- The doctor was very rude.

- No one told us our father was dying of kidney failure. We would have done things differently if we'd known.

- Seems like someone could have at least read the medical record. We did not feel like they knew my son. Very stressful.

- Care provided was essentially protocol-driven with very little personal attention.

- Some nurses were competent, others were absolutely negligent in care provided (e.g., changing IV without gloves), and within 24 hours an infection set in.

- Left side rail of bed down after brain surgery, and my mother fell out of the bed in the ICU.

One family member described the problems they experienced in scheduling their two-year-old son, who was diagnosed with autism. Their son needed an MRI, and they encountered very poor coordination in the scheduling process. The lack of care and attention in the scheduling process resulted in their feeling mistrust for the quality of the care itself. Our survey landed in her inbox while she was right in the middle of a maddeningly frustrating process. She responded:

My son is an ongoing patient in a rehab center. Meeting the Pediatric Neurologist went well. The next step, scheduling my 2-year-old son for his first MRI, went very poorly. No one gave me directions in how to prepare. I called multiple times, and each person gave me their "best guess," and no two people gave the same information. I was told to come 15 minutes prior, 30 minutes prior, and 2 hours prior to the procedure. I still don't know which is right. As of Friday at 3pm no one had called me with any information so I moved his Monday procedure date to Wednesday, and still I have heard from no one. When I called and shared my concern, I was told they don't know what's going on— that there must be a communication breakdown somewhere but they don't know where. Not only was my initial scheduling request not heard, I also told them my son cannot understand speech nor is he able to speak, so if he cannot eat or drink before the MRI he needs to be the 1st one scheduled that day or he will have multiple meltdowns and will be very stressed as he will not be able to understand why he can't have any food or water until 3:00 in the afternoon. Even after I explained this, he was still placed as the last patient of the day! And he is 2. I need someone to reach me ASAP as this has greatly increased our stress and I still have no directions on how to prepare.

This is a prime example of the suffering that can be caused by systemic misattunement. This respondent also told us that no more than a few days prior to this experience, she had received her son's life-changing diagnosis of autism in a letter, rather than a personal phone call from the physician. The mother said that she liked their doctor and had faith in him, but their experience with the process and the broader team was so abysmal that they lost trust in the whole system.

Survey Responses: "Moments of Frustration or Anger about Loved One's Care"

Sixty-seven percent of respondents indicated they have experienced moments of anger and frustration during their loved one's episode of care. Their reported experiences fall into four themes:

1. Lack of compassion

2. Lack of attunement

3. Not listening to or not believing the patient or family

4. Unexpected outcomes without support and resolution

These themes are consistent with literature that describes anger in patients and families being associated with lack of nursing presence and availability, lack of attention to patients' physical and/or psychological needs, and failure of caregivers to recognize the uniqueness and wholeness of individuals (Koloroutis & Trout, 2012; Plaas, 2002; Shattell & Hogan, 2005).

Lack of Compassion

Compassionate care is the highest priority for family members. It bears noting, however, that compassionate care is not limited to evidence of attunement and genuine concern from individual caregivers. The processes and structures of the organization can also convey compassion or the lack of it. Compassionate care includes coordinated teamwork, with the patient experiencing that she is at the center of the team's focus.

When family members witness the absence of key things such as attunement, caring actions, attention to privacy and dignity, attending to comfort, and working as a team on behalf of their loved one, they may experience helplessness and fear. They worry about their loved one's safety. They worry about their loved one's dignity. It is a short path from these very sensible worries to frustration and anger. It is within this context that a family member may ultimately be labeled as "demanding" by some members of the health care team. As we listen to our respondents' stories, we can easily see how one event builds on another and creates a pattern of frustration and ultimately the loss of trust. The following two examples bring this to life. The first is an emergency department experience, and the second took place in a long-term care setting. In both situations, family members advocated for their loved one's care.

Compassionate care is not limited to evidence of attunement and genuine concern from individual caregivers. The processes and structures of the organization can also convey compassion or the lack of it.

> The care provided was essentially protocol driven with very little personal attention. It was mechanical with very little interest in us. The response to various needs was either slow or didn't happen. There was inconsistent communication between primary care physician and family. The total team seemed broken in terms of communication and long term planning. As the patient's family member I had to ask for a team meeting, as no one seemed to be in charge of the care. The hospitalists changed with the shifts, and often the hand-off was not there. As a family we received different messages on the trajectory of care and next steps. It was a very unsettling experience. We were not a part of the care team.

My husband is in a nursing home due to a stroke. I became angry when there was such an apparent lack of sensitivity to his basic human needs (e.g., lack of privacy during bathing, rough handling of him when moving, not noticing that his feet were touching the end of the bed, not thoroughly washing him after being incontinent, and speaking to him harshly). When I saw the CNA placing soiled linens on his overbed table, touching the privacy curtain, the handle to bathroom, the water pitcher etc., with soiled gloves, I stopped her, pointed out my concerns, then asked to speak with her in the presence of the supervising LPN. I discussed each issue, what needed to improve, and why. I also talked to an administrator about the situation, which was not an isolated occurrence, and about my expectations as to what needed to improve and my suggestions as to how to proceed.

Lack of Attunement

A lack of attunement was perceived by the family members we surveyed when clinicians exhibited "disinterest, poor communication, and distracted presence." One family member had a sense that "I don't matter to you." There was a perception that the health care worker was simply doing a job, completing tasks, and not concerned about the family members or their wellbeing. Disconnection and ineffective or truncated communications convey lack of care and concern and demonstrate what it means to be misattuned. Here are more comments from our survey:

- Caregivers did not even pretend to be engaged.

- Caregivers did not introduce themselves or know the plan.

- No one was communicating with me, and no one seemed like they could help.

- The lack of communication angered me on behalf of my mother.

- Some of the nurses seemed less interested in our concerns for our loved one's health and more concerned with finishing their shift.

- It was frustrating when we asked legitimate questions, and it seemed as if we were bothering the nurse. It was more frustrating when the nursing staff found out that I am a nurse as well, and their attitude of disinterest turned quickly to annoyance.

Not Listening to or Not Believing the Patient or Family

Responses to our survey suggest that not being listened to is a very common complaint from patients and family members alike. People who do not feel heard and understood often either put more (and often louder) effort into feeling heard and understood, or they withdraw efforts to communicate. Either way, the potential is high for missing information that would more fully inform the care. Family members who feel dismissed or shut out, or witness their loved one not being listened to, are likely to become highly vigilant and mistrusting. The experience of not being listened to was reported in our survey as a key factor in feeling angry during the health care experience:

Family members who feel dismissed or shut out, or witness their loved one not being listened to, are likely to become highly vigilant and mistrusting.

- When we were in the emergency department, I wasn't heard when I voiced my concerns about my son's undiagnosed second fracture (collarbone). I'm an orthopedic nurse, and I've seen fractures of that nature for the last seven years. The fracture was diagnosed a week later at the clinic.

- The discharge doctor acted as though we knew nothing. She had answers to questions we didn't care about, and the questions we were concerned about, she ignored.

- We were not listened to by the doctor. We told him that this sudden severe depression seemed to be a rapid onset, triggered by prescribed steroids. The doctor said, "No, it shouldn't do that." Even though we saw a clear connection, he simply dismissed us. It took a conversation with a pharmacist by my brother to get them to even consider the possibility.

- I felt angry about the failure of the health professionals to listen to the patient. There was a failure to be interested in my mother's perspective, report of symptoms, and a failure to provide guidance about the best way to provide care for herself.

- It was frustrating to relay my concerns and have them be ignored, because I know what my loved one's "norm" is. Then to be called late at night to be told my loved one had declined . . .

- I felt very upset when the nurses did not believe my daughter's description of pain and took no definitive action. They kept adjusting the dosage and then saying we will wait and see. This went on for 24 hours postsurgery until we became very upset and demanded a pain consult. Only then were we listened to, and as a result of the consultation, the medication was changed and her pain relieved. Our daughter's suffering would not have gone on for so long if the nurses would have really listened and believed her.

Unexpected Outcomes without Support and Resolution

When family members learn that their loved one suffered an unexpected medical outcome due to a complication or unanticipated change in status, the family experiences distress. When an unexpected outcome is not clearly acknowledged to the family, including full and honest disclosure if something went awry, they are left to struggle with emotions ranging from guilt to rage to abandonment. In the survey, a daughter described feeling angry about the tragic outcome of a routine procedure:

My father never woke up from the biopsy. After several days we had to make a choice to take him off all supportive measures. The doctors don't know why he didn't wake up after the procedure.

Certainly, it would be very hard to have your loved one not awaken after a biopsy, and anger—a common expression of loss and grief— would be a normal human response (Koloroutis & Trout, 2012). One is left to wonder, however, in reading her simple description, whether there could have been more done to help her reconcile and cope with this unexpected loss.

Another daughter wrote about not knowing that her father was experiencing kidney failure and that he was dying. She describes taking her father to his medical appointments, with no one telling her that his kidneys were failing.

> It may have been the result of health care confidentiality, but I had no idea my father was terminally ill. I thought I was caring for him because of an injury due to a fall, and about a week before he was hospitalized I accompanied him to a visit with his kidney specialist to learn that his kidneys were failing. No one had mentioned this during the six weeks I was caring for him.

His ultimate death came as an unexpected outcome. She continues to struggle with why she was not more involved and informed. She was his primary caregiver.

Survey Response: "These are What We Would Like to See Caregivers Do"

We asked the respondents to choose from the following list of behaviors the two that they would consider most important in the care of their loved one:

- Be present and attuned when giving care.

- Listen to and respect my loved one's thoughts and feelings.

- Follow through: Do what you say you will do, and inform us that you have.

- Keep us informed about what is happening and what is going to happen.

- Treat my loved one with dignity and respect.

- Be interested in what my loved one is telling you about what he or she needs.

- Work with my loved one to control pain and alleviate suffering.

- Touch my loved one gently and with care.

The response chosen most often (68%) was, "Keep us informed about our loved one's care."

Second was the importance of being present and attuned (36%). Two respondents said the following:

> Sit down and talk to me, even if you only have 1–2 minutes. Listen to what I say. Be present, curious. Don't *know* everything, and please do not act like I am a bother and an intrusion on your day. This is a person I love. I know her, and I can help.

> It is nearly impossible to actually select just two behaviors from the list as they are all important. I want my loved one to be cared about as a human being; if this occurs I believe her needs will be met.

While the highest priority was keeping the patient and family informed, respondents also stressed the importance of the health care team members keeping each other informed on behalf of the patient.

> Inform one another. My daughter's doctor, PT, and OT don't practice at the same location so they don't have a chance to discuss her case, but it would be helpful if they at least shared records.

> It would be great if the same questions were not asked repeatedly by different people on the health care team. It makes us feel like they don't share information with each other, and our daughter has to repeat the same information over and over. It makes us wonder if anyone is listening or cares enough to pass our information along.

Survey Response: "Deep Moments of Appreciation for Our Loved One's Care"

Eighty-six percent of the respondents said they experienced moments of deep appreciation. These moments provided comfort and solace to families who found themselves at their loved one's side in times of trouble. This is one of many stories told in response to the question about whether the respondents experienced moments of appreciation for a loved one's care.

My mom was going through chemotherapy once a week for four months. I was pregnant at the time and we drove two hours one way to get her to the best treatment center. I didn't miss a treatment. I rearranged my work schedule to be there. I gave birth to my daughter midway through the treatments. The team in the outpatient clinic let me bring my baby girl to the appointments while my mom was getting chemo. We were told my mom may not make it as breast cancer with lymphoma has a grim prognosis. The staff was so welcoming and accommodating to everyone who wanted to be with my mom during this time. They let Mom hold Maria, her granddaughter, during her treatments . . . the staff was awesome, they really looked out for my mom's mental and emotional wellbeing and she needed that. They scheduled her appointments to be in the large treatment room and blocked space as there were usually ten or more of us. They let all of us in that room to laugh, cry, and talk to Mom during her treatments. This meant so much to us. It was an amazing experience. The good news is that the grim picture turned around. My mom is still alive 15 years later.

The stories of appreciation reflect many moments of therapeutic connection. Not surprisingly, the primary source of appreciation for family members was witnessing their loved ones being treated with dignity, compassion, and competence. They felt the caregiving team "had their back," that the team was genuinely committed to their loved one's wellbeing. The moments of deep appreciation described by the respondents appear in Figure 4.3 on the following two pages, organized according to the therapeutic practices—attuning, wondering, following, and holding—which they best exemplify. We were struck by how beautifully the language of the family respondents brings the therapeutic practices to life.

Attuning	She was present; was not going through a routine.
	The caregiver (nurse or physician) was tuned in … there was somebody home … not going through the motions …
	The nurse was so compassionate; showed concern.
	The care team was invested in my husband.
	They took the time to be with us.
	The pharmacist paused and listened … was not dismissive.
	They joined us; very attentive to me and my adult children.
	A nurse noticed our distress.
	The staff had a deep understanding of the needs of my critically ill infant and my needs as his mother.
	They seemed to understand my needs, sometimes before I did. It calmed me.
	They invited my input and acknowledged that I had important information that only a family member could contribute.
Wondering and Following	The anesthesiologist approached my daughter with respect, kindness, patience, and genuine curiosity … my daughter visibly relaxed in her care.
	She asked questions, paused, and listened.
	The physician was open and curious.
	The nurse wanted to know what I was seeing; she recognized that I had important information about my mother.
	He asked and listened.
	He cared enough to find out who my boyfriend was as a person.

Holding	The nurse kept us informed; even stopped on her way out to give us an update.
	My mother was in a coma, and I observed a staff member gently touching her shoulder and speaking gently and compassionately to her.
	The nurse embraced our grieving group.
	The staff called my loved one by name.
	The whole team was concerned for her comfort, pain relief, positioning in bed.
	He used reassuring words and a warm and gentle tone.
	The staff honored my father [a veteran] after his death by draping him in a flag and standing quietly by as his body was moved to the morgue; very moving and unexpected.
	They let us take our time in making our decision to stop treatment. They didn't judge us or rush us.

Figure 4.3: Patients' and Families' Words of Appreciation, Organized According to the Therapeutic Practice They Express

Moving Forward

One of the things that became clear to us through the survey responses was how little it took for people to feel held. The families were asking for very little—usually for some acknowledgment of their difficulty. Here again are the words of Marvelyne Engel to crystalize how easily connections can be made with the families of our patients.

If you take a bit of time just to relate to the family and assure the family that you're working together, with them, not against them . . . that moment of insider advice when you say, "The good coffee's on the 3rd floor" . . . makes such a difference in how we're going to respond to you and receive help from you. (Creative Health Care Management, 2013)

Marvelyne is talking about feeling seen as a person and how meaningful an extremely small gesture can be. The words were, "The good coffee's on the 3rd floor," but the sentiment was, "I see you, I see the state you're in, and we're in this together."

A vital part of advancing a relationship-based culture is helping the families of patients feel held in our care—helping them to feel as though we are truly in it together. It is a characteristic of RBC organizations that at every touch point, care remains at a consistently high level. Consistently caring for families is one of the things that makes a major difference to your patients' overall sense of wellbeing and security. The feeling that "we're all on the same side" comes not just from individuals and teams; it comes also from processes and structures. For this reason, we offer the reflection tool below, in Figure 4.4, to assist you in designing your systems to optimize quality, safety, and the patient experience by involving and supporting families in patient care.

Part One: Group Reflection	
What is our current state of family involvement?	What do we believe about families and care?
	What do we view as the benefits of family involvement? What do we consider burdens?
	How easy are our processes for obtaining permission to share patient information with family members?
	Are our beliefs and practices consistent with current evidence on family engagement? If not, what do we need to change?
	Do we have a family-friendly lounge?
	In the clinic, are there chairs for family members?
	How easy is wayfinding in our facility? Do all members of our organization stop and help lost-looking family members find what they are looking for, accompanying them to the destination?
What is our vision for family involvement?	What will our care for families look like?
	What do our families tell us matters most in our care provision?
	In what ways do our processes facilitate care? Based on family input, what are specific opportunities for improvement?
	What needs to change in our beliefs? In our actions?

Part Two: Taking Action

What are we willing to do to involve families as partners?	What is our commitment to patients' families?
	What key actions do we need to take to move us toward our vision for family involvement?
	What written materials would help our team to actualize our commitment to families?
	What quality or lean processes do we need to institute to improve our care?
	What actions do we need to take to include the family's input at key times (e.g., handoffs, admission, discharge, moments of crisis, etc.)?
	How does our website support our vision for families? What needs to change?
	How do we speak about families in our policies and signage? Is the language welcoming? Does it convey the view that families are welcomed as partners in care?
	Do we have a consistent, dedicated section within the electronic health record for all care providers to use to share personal information about the patient's family care partners?
	Do we have a patient and family advisory group? What would it take to create one? How can we partner with the advisory group to strengthen and improve care?

Figure 4.4: Questions for Group Reflection and Action

As we reflect, rethink, redesign, and realign our systems to more intentionally work with and care for families, let us keep in mind that their needs are simple: They want to be seen and heard; they want to be informed and to understand what is expected of them; they want their loved one to receive the best possible care; and they want to be a part of the caring process. Families hold important insights into what would constitute optimal care for their loved ones because they know them best. As health care providers striving for excellence, we need those closest to the patient to be part of our team and should do everything in our power to welcome them into the care and healing of their loved ones.

Summary of Key Thoughts

- If the inclusion of the family is to be central to the care experience, the health care team must intentionally involve the family in the patient's care and provide therapeutic support to the family.

- Research has confirmed that the presence and participation of family members and friends as partners in care provides cost savings, enhances the patient and family experience of care, improves management of chronic and acute illnesses, enhances continuity of care, and prevents hospital readmissions.

- The onus is upon us as health care providers to provide information, care, and loving attention, alongside and in partnership with whatever family members the patient deems to be the primary family contacts.

- It is essential for people in all care settings to examine their beliefs about the role of family members in the care of the patient. If these beliefs go unexamined, they harden into biases, and biases shut down curiosity and therapeutic connection.

- Family members report being very pleased with care when caregivers are present and attuned, when communication is thorough and consistent, and when it is apparent to them that the team is working together on behalf of their loved one.

- Common reasons for family dissatisfaction with care include inadequate or unskilled communication, ineffective teamwork, lack of individualized attention, and lack of clinical competence—all of which compromise quality and safety.

Reflection

- What are examples of language commonly used in your care environment that reveal something, positive or negative, about how families are thought of? If it's negative language you identified, what language could replace it?

- What would it take for you to "pause and get curious" the next time a family member of a patient did or said something unkind to you, a member of your team, or the patient? What do you think might happen if you paused and got curious?

- Reflect on a situation in which you received vital information from a family member that you could not have received from any other source.

- Considering that the loved ones of seriously ill patients are in non-ordinary states, how might this inform your care?

SECTION TWO
Leadership

Most important of all, "love leadership" is not just a better way to lead but a more fulfilling way to live. At the end of the day, love leaders know they have lived their lives with integrity; developed authentic, lasting relationships; and enhanced every environment they have been in by their presence. That alone makes it all worthwhile.

BILL GEORGE

CHAPTER FIVE

Loving Leaders Advance Healing Cultures

JAYNE FELGEN AND PAMELA SCHAID

How often do discussions of leadership include the word *love*? Whether it has been intentionally placed to the side or simply assumed that there is no place for love in leadership, we find that words like *loving* have not typically led the list of characteristics that describe an outstanding leader. Words like *strategic, visionary, analytical, fiscally responsible,* and *team-focused* might top the list, but somehow the seat of our humanity, the willingness to be guided by love, doesn't usually make the list. Still, when we reflect on those positional leaders we've known who stand out as exemplars, we do not have to look too deeply to see the love. It was there. You could feel it in their actions, interactions, values, and purpose. When we think of those leaders, words such as *purposeful, attentive, authentic, trustworthy, patient, vulnerable, kind, generous, humble, respectful, sincere, caring,* and *unselfish* come right to mind. Love led the way; most of us just haven't named it as such. In our work as nurses, executive leaders, and consultants in health care, we have been privileged to witness those who lead and manage in ways that help to advance the cultures of their organizations into what they want them to be—cultures that help people heal, not just recover. In this chapter we share lessons from their leadership.

What Is Loving Leadership?

Love as an element of leadership is not a new concept. Discussions of loving leadership can be traced back to the ancient Tao, which equates love with leading by serving. The servant leader shares power, puts the needs of others first, and helps people develop and perform as competently as possible (Greenleaf, 1991). Loving leadership is a key ingredient in recipes for leaders aspiring to advance a more positive healing culture within their organizations. Inspired leaders who love what they do and the people with whom they do it, inspire others to greatness. We have long held that successful organizations thrive when their leaders know and believe that there is a leader in every chair. We now also assert that the presence of love at all levels of the organization is a driving force in achieving quality, safety, and exemplary patient-centered experiences.

Inspired leaders who love what they do and the people with whom they do it, inspire others to greatness.

Loving leadership is marked by deep affection and caring for those with whom we work and lead. It is a deep devotion with feelings of caring and respect. It involves nurturing, supporting growth and development, wanting the best for each person, and desiring to help people identify their gifts, talents, and strengths. Love in leadership means truly caring about each person, celebrating successes, as well as having empathy in times of struggle. It includes releasing judgment and forgiving past difficulties. It means being fully present in our interactions.

We have been told that "love and work do not go together" (hooks [sic], 2000). Love is understood as soft and intangible—something that cannot be measured—and yet it is the glue which holds relationships together and inspires commitment to a shared mission. Love in leadership is about changing the lens through which we view our workplace world. It is about empowerment of self and others, and it is about a willingness to be vulnerable, which allows us to connect at a deeper level.

What We Learned in Conversation with Eight Loving Leaders

As we prepared this chapter, we had the privilege of meeting with eight leaders, not all of whom work in health care, but all of whom lead with love. They allowed us to record our conversations so that their words could be included in this chapter. We were honored to meet with these remarkable leaders:

Peter Block is the author or coauthor of eight books on organizational development, community building, and civic engagement.

Glenn Costie is CEO of the Dayton VA Medical Center in Dayton, Ohio.

Mary Del Guidice is CNO of Pennsylvania Hospital and assistant dean for Clinical Practice and senior fellow of the Center for Health Policy and Outcomes Research at the University of Pennsylvania School of Nursing in Philadelphia, Pennsylvania.

Matt Marchbanks is the director of business development at Sodexo.

Anne McNamara is former president of Galen College of Nursing and current principal at McNamara Solutions, a leadership-based health care consulting firm.

Tim Porter-O'Grady is a clinical professor and leadership scholar at The Ohio State University and the author of 21 books on shared governance, professional practice, and leadership.

Rosanne Raso is CNO at New York–Presbyterian/Weill Cornell Medical Center and the executive editor of *Nursing Management*.

Rear Admiral Michael Weahkee is CEO of the Phoenix Indian Medical Center in Phoenix, Arizona, Indian Health Service, and Assistant Surgeon General in the U.S. Public Health Service.

As we examined the transcripts of our conversations, we looked for commonalities among how these eight people think about love in leadership and how they seek to express it in their work. We discovered this:

- Each leader had been mentored, formally or informally, by a loving leader, and each felt compelled to pay that mentoring forward. We call this a *thread of love* connecting generations of loving leaders.

- Most of the leaders mentioned that they prized authenticity, vulnerability, and humility in other leaders and aspired to demonstrate it in their own leadership.

- All demonstrated recognition of the interconnectedness of all people, using language such as, "We're all in this together."

The Thread of Love (or If You See Something, Say Something)

When we asked each of the loving leaders we spoke with about the leaders who made a difference in their early lives and careers, a theme emerged that was 100% consistent among them. Each loving leader spoke of someone having seen something in them that they hadn't seen in themselves. The best term for what they saw is *potential,* but it showed up more specifically as integrity, passion, excellent performance, and/or a high level of commitment to the work. While each leader could be described, in his or her early career, as "eager to succeed," their definitions of success were often humble, tending to be a version of, "I just wanted to do a good job." Mary Del Guidice, now a chief nursing officer, had a very clear vision of herself being a bedside nurse for her entire career, but when opportunities to make a broader difference were presented to her, she found enough of them irresistible that she ended up in a leadership position and eventually as an executive leader. Someone saw in her the ability to do more and have a broader effect. Her leadership ability was something she hadn't seen in herself, but when it was reflected back to her by someone she trusted and admired, she believed it.

Some version of this story was told to us by each of the eight leaders we spoke to, and it always had an additional component: All of these leaders described their own practices of seeing the best qualities of others and reflecting those qualities back to them. Interestingly, not everyone saw this as an act of love, but once we named it for them, there was consensus that even though they hadn't necessarily intended to express love, seeing the good in others and naming

Seeing the good in others and naming it is an inherently loving act.

it is an inherently loving act. This "naming the good in others" draws people closer together and helps people feel safe, because it provides evidence that they are not merely seen, but that they are *deeply* seen by someone they regard as a person of substance. As Peter Block said, "A love-based leader sees the gifts and capacities in people."

Perhaps because these leaders had someone see in them the right skill set and temperament for leadership, they are good at seeing it in others. Here's Glenn Costie talking about an early mentor:

> I didn't realize it at the time, but one of my mentors frequently picked me for difficult assignments in which an organization or department was failing, and it was my job to turn it around . . . This has happened through many parts of my career, and I realize now that they were all situations in which there was strife and conflict, and the people were feeling abused. They all needed love, and that was part of what we provided, even though we never said the word or even thought about it. You can't help feeling compassion when you see how people are suffering. You want to provide healing for the people and the organization, and that's a loving impulse.

Would any given leader have been able to heal the abuses Costie spoke of? What about someone with more experience or a more impressive track record than Costie had back then? Not necessarily. When an organization or department is failing, it's very hard on the staff. They get disheartened and start to doubt their abilities. They may fear, quite reasonably, that they will lose their jobs. Sometimes, along with the necessary improvements in systems and processes, they also need love. So why does it feel slightly dangerous to say so? Why does it feel perfectly safe to say, "We're going to need to make some changes around here, and you're probably not going to like some of them," but it feels more than a little risky to say, "When I look at this organization, this staff, my heart is full of love"?

We are inspired to call this legacy of seeing the good in others and naming it a *thread of love* because it makes its way, seemingly without exception, from one generation of loving leaders to the next. What was clear in our conversations is that these leaders all had the benefit of this loving practice and that they integrated it into their own way of being. As Mary Del Guidice told us, "I wanted to be like my CNO. I wanted to be able to make anyone I came into contact with feel as special as she made me feel." But why was this pattern so consistent? We found ourselves wondering if the magic in this practice is that it actually transforms the receiver—that perhaps a person who feels unseen and not valued is fundamentally different from a person who feels seen and valued. Perhaps when someone you respect and admire sees something of value in you and says so, something is activated in you, and perhaps a characteristic of that *something* is that, since you cannot pay the favor back, you are compelled to pay it forward.

For loving leaders, there is no downside to developing the next generation. Admiral Michael Weahkee shared this:

> The risk of not developing the next generation is that you have underdeveloped resources, and you'll have to take on more yourself. When I develop others, eventually they will get to the point where they can develop the next generation. They'll have the knowledge, education, and modeling of how to continue. It won't just stop with me. I feel like I have a personal responsibility to pass it on ... to take what was given to me and share it with others and support others. I have the capacity to teach more than one—as many as are willing.

This shows a generosity of spirit, but perhaps more impressively, it shows a generosity of time. When questioned about his capacity to mentor larger numbers of people, Weahkee continued:

> I do feel I have a very large capacity to mentor others. Even if the number of people I mentor now quadruples, it would be manageable. There's definitely the capacity to meet and spend an hour every month or so with however many people would like to come and do so. There are ways to reach larger audiences, but you can't overemphasize the value of the one-on-one relationship.

This expression of generosity of time and spirit came from a man who later shared, with great vulnerability, that his difficult beginnings made his experience with his own mentors mean more to him than he could express. Someone reached into his life and saw his leadership potential.

Again, Weahkee:

> I didn't have a lot of support growing up. If it's not there, and then suddenly you do have somebody helping you out, it's all the more powerful.

Loving leaders remember that patients and families are not the only people in their care. They see themselves also as trustees of their staff's wellbeing. One of the ways Mary Del Guidice has found to show her love for her staff is to believe in them. She shared an acknowledgment she received from one of her nurses on the day of our conversation. It said, "Thank you for believing in us and for not leaving us when you realized that we weren't what you thought we were." She's not only thanking Mary for loving the staff; she's acknowledging that Mary's love is unconditional. It's no surprise that she sees that love, expressed as belief in the abilities of others, spreading throughout the organization as well:

Loving leaders remember that patients and families are not the only people in their care. They see themselves as trustees of their staff's wellbeing.

> I constantly hear my team say, "I know this nurse is up to the task, I believe in her, she can do this." I think that kind of belief in people is a force that can move mountains. People can feel it when you believe in them, just like when my CNO believed in me. I remember thinking, "Wow, I feel like I've got wings!"

This thread of love also makes leaders throw their protégées into the deep end, sometimes before they realize they're ready. Here's Anne McNamara:

> One of my mentors, Dr. Lillian Goodman, came to me and said that there had been an unfortunate death on the board of directors and that she had put my name forward to sit on the board. There were some practical reasons that I was a fit, but I was in my 20s and was stunned by the idea. In meetings, the chair of the Board of Directors would turn to me and say, "So Anne, what are your thoughts on that?" It wasn't just about giving everybody a turn to talk either. I was the voice of the staff nurses, and the board needed to understand how

the staff nurses would be impacted. I was the voice of thousands and thousands of staff nurses out there.

Perhaps loving leaders take chances on others because loving leaders took chances on them.

Authenticity and Vulnerability

What we have just described as seeing the best in others and naming it could, we realize, be done as a tactic, much like the now discredited leadership tactic of sandwiching negative feedback between two pieces of positive feedback. Even if people didn't detect the pattern, they could tell they were being managed as employees rather than connected with as people.

Poet David Whyte (2010) identifies vulnerability as a "core human competence." It is a strength, an ally. Brené Brown (2010) points out that vulnerability is an important foundation of love. Lashley and colleagues (1994) write about how vulnerability is inherent within our professional identity and is necessary for growth. Every day, health care workers come face to face with ethical dilemmas, complex problems requiring complex solutions, and the discomfort of not knowing all the answers. We are continually confronted with experiences of fear, pain, risk, and suffering. Lashley and colleagues (1994) wondered whether creating environments that honor this vulnerability by modeling it, accepting it, being gentle with it, and unconditionally supporting it would create "holding" environments that might "[nurture] a new language, a lived language of vulnerability" (p. 48), in which we acknowledge its continuous presence in our lives.

Clearly, unless the practice of seeing the best in people and naming it is authentic, it risks being seen as insincere and manipulative. The reason naming the good in others has been so effective for these leaders is that it's an authentic expression of what they see. Here's a story from Mary Del Guidice that illustrates the benefit of authenticity in leadership:

> When I was a kid, my dad was an executive at NBC television, and he would take us to his office once a year, at Christmastime. We would walk around 30 Rockefeller Plaza in Manhattan, and I remember being so struck that he knew everybody. He knew the cameraman's

name, he knew the name of the guy who was sweeping the floor, he knew the newscaster's name. And with every person he would stop. "Oh, Bob, thanks for doing a great job" or "Rose! It's good to see you! How's your son?" And I just couldn't get over the fact that he knew everyone and they knew him, and they were thanking him and he was thanking them—I was so inspired by that. As a child at home, I'd imagined what being an executive would be like, and I pictured my dad in a big office moving papers around and talking on the phone and making decisions. But then I'd be with him at work and think, "This is just my dad being my dad." I knew the way he loved us at home, and he was that same loving guy at work.

This is a story of a man who went on to be president of Operations and Technical Services for the entire NBC network. We realize how unlikely it is that the people who hired him were specifically looking for a leader who exhibited authenticity, but fortunately for them, that's what they got. It also took no small measure of vulnerability for this leader to show up as his authentic self in such a high-powered position in such a high-pressure industry. He could have hidden behind the persona of a strong, decisive, powerful leader who ruled with an iron fist. Instead, he showed up as who he really was: a strong, decisive, powerful leader who cared deeply about everyone in the organization and did his best to provide an environment in which everyone could thrive. He was ahead of his time. As was perhaps *not* true several decades ago, vulnerability and authenticity are no longer seen as liabilities in leaders. Even people in very high-powered positions can succeed by truly being who they are, rather than projecting a false sense of hypercompetence. People tend to work hard for leaders who really see them and acknowledge their dedication and good work. It creates an environment in which people feel connected to a shared purpose, even if, as in the case of a television network, that purpose is to provide a profitable consumer product.

Unless the practice of seeing the best in people and naming it is authentic, it risks being seen as insincere and manipulative.

In health care, we have the additional benefit of a larger mission to guide us, and that larger mission provides a standing invitation for leaders to lead with both vulnerability and authenticity. Because of the nature of our work, most of our "customers" are in a vulnerable state—they're compromised either temporarily or permanently. They're in non-ordinary states, needful of greater human connection. They need us to demonstrate that we're attuned to them—that we see them and that we're working together to weave a web of protection around them. This web of protection can do the job of reassuring patients and families, however, only if it is created by people exhibiting some degree of authenticity and vulnerability. The loving leaders we spoke with did not call out their own authenticity—not even as something they aspired to. Instead, they pointed to authenticity in those who had mentored them, and they effortlessly demonstrate it every day. Here again is Mary Del Guidice:

> I think it really is those who just stand up there, full hearted, put it all out there, that people connect with, they want to follow, they admire, they love back. I think you can get through the tough days with those kinds of leaders. It's the same with leaders as it is with clinical nurses. How many times did we as nurses check the schedule to see who we were working with? You knew you were going to have a good day if you were working with the nurse who really cared the most. It didn't matter if you had two sheets to share and all the meals were cold and half the team called in sick; if you were working with that one nurse, it was going to be a great day. I cared about being that kind of nurse, and I care about being that kind of leader.

We're All in This Together

The loving leaders we spoke with all expressed a sense of oneness with their staff. They spoke in ways that indicated that they were simultaneously accountable for the whole and inexorably "in it" with everyone in the organization. Here is Peter Block:

> The world treats leadership as an individual act, but it's a communal act. We say that an individual has to find his or her voice, but it's not so

much a voice to speak up against the system; it's finding the courage to speak together.

Loving leaders also have a sense that their responsibility for their team's wellbeing extends beyond the walls of the organization. They know that what happens on somebody's 12-hour shift is a pretty small fraction of that person's whole life. Here is Anne McNamara:

> If somebody gets a call from school and his kid is sick, I'm on it. I ask, "What's hanging out there—what do we need covered? We'll do what we need to do, but you go and do what you need to do as a parent." If someone has a mom or dad who's older and might be sick or actively dying, I'll sit someone down and say, "You need to go and be with your dad; you need to leave and just focus on family right now." I believe that's one of the ways I show love.

McNamara continues, referencing a quote by John Hope Bryant that we'd provided as inspiration for our discussion:

> Love releases energy, and employees deserve to have energy left over at the end of the day for their partners, their kids, and their communities. (Bryant, 2009)

It's important to note that this story was *not* followed by any sort of caveat such as, "It takes a lot out of the rest of us, but we do it." Instead it was spoken of as though helping someone in need (dare we say a loved one in need?) is an honor.

One of the most beautiful stories we heard about a leader who was a natural partner came from Rosanne Raso. When we asked her to recall mentors who had affected her throughout her career, she pointed to someone who reported to her rather than someone who was in a position to provide her with guidance or advancement:

> Jose Hernandez's approach was, "Okay, team, let's get together as a group. We can do this together. We can help each other. What do we need from each other?" And later, when whatever initiative they were working on would be rolled out, it was with the same spirit. We'd collaborated, had the same clear goals, we'd shared a purpose, and

people felt good about what we created. He's an example of what happens when love meets practicality.

What Rosanne Raso learned from Jose Hernandez was that it is just plain true that we really are all in this together. The togetherness wasn't something he made happen. In fact, we believe it's never something someone makes happen. Instead, it's a truth that is revealed by loving, insightful leaders who are tuned in to the interconnectedness of all of the people they cross paths with. Here's a story from Tim Porter-O'Grady that amplifies that reality:

I had done a lot of work in the 1980s starting the concept of shared governance, and in the '90s I was doing a presentation at an organization, and a person came up to me whom I'd never met before. She just wanted to tell me that she'd heard me speak ten years ago and that I'd had an unbelievable impact on her life. It was a compliment, but it sent me into a mental tailspin. I thought, "What if the real purpose of my life had been conveying whatever I'd conveyed to her in that earlier presentation?" In the hours and days that followed, I thought a lot about it, and then I sort of turned it over and looked at the dark side. What if there were also moments when I had done or said something that facilitated the "dark force," if you will. So it became very important to me to have integrity in how I formed my life, my work, my relationships.

Porter-O'Grady understands that we are all interconnected, whether we pay that reality any mind or not, and it created in him a heightened sense of responsibility. Because he was up in front of people and seen as an authority, he knew that his words carried weight and that he owed it to the world to be careful with them. It's clear also that he sees himself as a "brother on the path" rather than as a person with all the answers:

The only thing you can do is to enable each other and engage each other along the way in the journey we're all on, in whatever way helps us move together on the trajectory. If I have a leadership role, I have an obligation to create a safe space for us to move forward together and to encourage it. I can enable your increasing ownership and opportunity in that journey, and that's what I'm going to do as long as I'm wearing the leadership hat.

Humility

When we asked our loving leaders about the personal qualities of their own mentors, they often pointed to humility as a defining characteristic that they both admired and aspired to. This is Matt Marchbanks:

> When I think about great leaders, great parents, great teachers, I think about technical expertise—they're all good at what they do— but for me, the differentiator is humility.

Humility is an expansion of the spirit of "we are all in this together." Humility begins with the belief by these loving leaders that they are serving the greater good, something bigger than themselves—that their work extends beyond their own accomplishments. Humble leaders value all of the contributions of each individual as a significant force in serving the greater good. Humble leaders are more focused on achieving the goals of the organization than on individual credit, and they can admit they don't have all the answers. As Peter Block said:

Humble leaders are more focused on achieving the goals of the organization than on individual credit.

> The best leaders I've known were the ones who sometimes said, "I don't know." They refused to take on the parental mantle. Loving leadership honors uncertainty.

Loving leaders also have the humility to learn from their mistakes. Humility allows a loving leader to be vulnerable and to take risks. Could it also be that humility plays a major part in a leader's resilience? This is Anne McNamara:

> It's important to have confidence in moving things forward even if there are failures along the way … just step back and look at it and learn from it.

She continues:

> Everybody brings their gifts and talents. I know what I'm good at, but I know there are others who are good at things I'm not good at, and those are the people I try to surround myself with. When I think about the people I've admired, they were all pillars of excellence in their particular area, and they also knew the boundaries of what they knew and what they didn't know.

Matt Marchbanks recognized humility in his mentors and sought to repeat it in his own leadership:

> The people who mentored me were so clear in who they were that they were comfortable being vulnerable with me; that allowed me to become a humble leader, to lead with humility even when I'm very clear and confident in what I'm doing.

Humility is about being with, working with, and partnering with others. Not one of us can go it alone. Humble leaders understand and recognize our shared humanity.

Goodness

The final characteristic of these loving leaders is one that we didn't mention earlier in this chapter because it is very hard to describe: All of the leaders we spoke with exhibited something we're reluctantly calling *goodness*. Our reluctance to name this is due to the fact that it's impossible to see into people's hearts, to know their true aims. Still, we cannot ignore that as we spoke with these leaders, there was a sense that it was important to each of them to be a good example, a good team member, a good person. They understood that the eyes of a great number of people were upon them, and they knew that, because of their elevated roles, they had a responsibility to demonstrate the highest level of integrity.

This brings us back to the fact that inherent in the work of health care is a sense of higher purpose. Because of the nature of the work we do, the organizations we create are like few other organizations, and our leaders must also be a cut above. Leaders in health care must excel not just in their ability to keep an organization profitable but in their ability to keep an organization pointed toward the less measurable aim of providing a space in which patients, families, and team members can consistently feel seen, valued, held, and cared for—a space in which they can feel loved. None of that can be faked. People feel seen only when we see them. They feel valued, held, and cared for only when we value, hold, and care for them. And they feel loved only when we love them.

Our findings do not support the idea that loving leaders can be mentored into being unless the seed of goodness is already there, begging to be watered. We do believe, however, that this seed of goodness is more common than not. It appears from our conversations that if there is a formula for loving leaders, it is this: When a healthy measure of self-questioning sits on a foundation of absolute clarity about the goodness of the mission, people respond positively. Here is Glenn Costie:

> I think to myself, "We're going to start moving down this path, and if we have to change midcourse, that's fine. I am not married to the one course of action." It's a matter of clarity; you can change course as needed because you're clear about the fact that you're moving toward the right goal.

We think we understand something about what it means to know what the "right" goal is. We think you know what's right when you're tapped into your own goodness.

One of the risks of exhibiting goodness is that you'll hear what Mary Del Guidice heard from a colleague, pretty early in her tenure, after she'd declared that what her staff needed most was love. This colleague said, "You know, Mary, those rainbows and lollipops may not work here." She walked out of the office thinking, "Well, I was hired with these rainbows and lollipops, so I'm going to keep going. I'll just have to figure out how to spread them in a different way."

We imagine that it is equally true that Mary would not have succeeded in just any organization and that not just any organization could have attracted Mary to work there. When a leader exhibits goodness during the interview process, you can bet she is looking for an organization in which it can flourish—where her seed of goodness will be watered and where she sees other seeds she can water.

From what we can tell, this sense of goodness is a source of power. This is Michael Weahkee:

> When I consider being a loving leader, it makes me feel like I have a purpose, and I have a reason. I feel that in my spine. That's what drives the perseverance and commitment in me: knowing that I can have an impact.

Our time with these loving leaders taught us that goodness is easy to spot if you're looking for it, which brings our summary of what we discovered in our conversations right back to where we started. "Seeing the best in others and naming it" has a lot in common with spotting the seeds of goodness in others and watering them. It's what loving leaders do, and that is a very fortunate thing.

The Four Practices of Loving Leaders: Attuning, Wondering, Following, and Holding

The four relational practices of attuning, wondering, following, and holding are actualized by most of us, quite naturally, in our best moments. The practices were originally identified through the observations Koloroutis and Trout (2012) made as they watched and deconstructed what behaviors people were most consistently exhibiting in successful interpersonal encounters (p. 3). When things went well and people appeared to feel seen and satisfied, attunement was always a factor, and wondering, following, and holding (either singularly or in myriad combinations) were evident as well. The loving leaders we spoke with demonstrated all four practices quite consistently, whether they were familiar with the names of the four practices or not.

We're going to share what attuning, wondering, following, and holding look like when leaders practice them, but first we want to say something about why effective leaders might choose to consciously engage in these practices. The practices do provide some "soft" advantages: It stands to reason that people will like you more if you attune, wonder, follow, and hold. The practices also make people more authentic, and authenticity, as we've said, has some profound advantages, not the least of which is that it fosters trust. However, we believe that the most compelling reason to consciously practice attuning, wondering, following, and holding is because they optimize every interaction and therefore every relationship. This is why the application of the four relational practices was chosen as one of the primary threads that runs through this book. The four practices are the how-to for healthy relationships. It is simply impossible to attune, wonder, follow, and hold without improving every relationship in which you practice these skills.

Attuning

Attuning is an intentional connection with others. It makes us curious about people, allows us to fully perceive the impact of our presence, and causes us to align ourselves with others. "Attunement means we see a person as a person rather than as an obstacle or an object or a labeled category" (Koloroutis & Trout, 2012, p. 67). These authors also tell us that compassion and empathy are deepened as a result of attuning to people. Leading with love means that we consistently attune to those with whom we interact. Our conscious attunement to others nurtures them (and the relationship itself), and it shows respect.

It is simply impossible to attune, wonder, follow, and hold without improving every relationship in which you practice these skills.

Focusing your attention on those you lead, one at a time or in groups, is an example of attuning. Attuning is simply "tuning in" to the person standing in front of you or the conversation happening around you. It is a way of being intentionally present that demonstrates respect for and value of the people you lead. Loving leaders—even those who have no awareness of the four relational practices—find themselves attuning to others because they have a genuine interest in the people with whom they share the honor and privilege of working. As we learned in our conversations, loving leaders attune enough to see skills, abilities, and potentials that those they're leading perhaps didn't see. While attunement can be a one-way action (i.e., you can attune to someone who cannot or will not attune to you), it leads most often to a mutual connection. Attuning to someone is an act of valuing, respecting, and acknowledging the importance of the person. Unless the person you're attuning to has strong barriers to receiving your attunement, he or she is likely to feel valued, respected, and seen in your presence.

Loving leaders attune to individuals, to teams, and to the systems they lead. When we attune within our teams we find our strengths, synergies, and shared vision. When we attune to systems we feel the power of the organization, which can be a great source of inspiration. Glenn Costie described his leadership team's attunement like this:

> Right now I have the most connected leadership team of any place I've ever worked, at any level in any role, and it has to be because of the culture we have here—it's because of Relationship-Based Care. That began on day one, and since then everything that we've been doing everywhere in the organization has been focused on building healthy relationships. The overall framework of our relationship and our love—I'll use that word now because I think we do all love each other—is that we really are a team. We're tuned in to each other, and we look out for one another.

Attunement, as you discovered in Chapter Three, is the doorway to human connection. It stands to reason, then, that it is among the most important leadership tools in existence.

Wondering

If you want trust to permeate your culture, cultivate the practice of wondering.

Wondering is defined as curiosity or genuine interest in another. In a therapeutic relationship, this is the practice that helps clinicians to relax their preconceived notions and to open all of their senses so they can discover what's going on with patients and families and/or stay in the mode of discovery until a way to care for (if not cure) the patient can be found. While that aspect of the practice of wondering applies beautifully to a leader's role as problem solver and strategist, there is another aspect to wondering that a leader can benefit from, perhaps a dozen times every day: The conscious decision to wonder keeps us from judging too quickly. Wondering helps leaders to assume the good intent of the people

Wondering helps leaders to assume the good intent of the people around them, particularly in times of upheaval or confusion.

around them, particularly in times of upheaval or confusion. This is an invaluable practice for every loving leader to embrace, and it is a phenomenal advantage to a culture when a leader can visibly spend time wondering with teams or the entire organization. The loving leaders we spoke with talked about how much they respected leaders who had the courage to admit they don't know everything. Peter Block clearly admires this quality:

> Not knowing is a relational asset. The best leaders I know were the ones who said, "I don't know. I don't need to know; together we'll figure it out."

He's talking about the relational asset of staying in a state of wonder longer—of not concluding so quickly. He expanded on this idea a few moments later:

> To me, love has to be associated with the willingness to support others' freedom, support others' purpose. One of the greatest acts of love I know is to believe that for every great idea, the opposite idea is also true.

The practice of wondering demonstrates that a leader is secure in not knowing, and the practice of inviting others to wonder with you is a visible demonstration of your eagerness to partner with the talented people in your organization.

Following

Following is about listening closely, following cues, and exploring. As Stephen Covey asserted in *The Seven Habits of Highly Effective People* (2013), seeking to understand before seeking to be understood is an essential practice for effective leaders. Attuning, wondering, and following are the means to understanding others.

The unfolding of someone else's story happens when we follow. As a leader, this practice optimizes your ability to stay informed while also providing others with the experience of

Following is either sincere and heartfelt, born of genuine interest, or it is not following.

being deeply listened to. This can be a transformational moment for people. When you lovingly listen to others, you give them the gift of your attention. It is vital, however, that this practice never be used as a technique. Following is either sincere and heartfelt, born of genuine interest, or it is not following.

Holding

Holding is a practice that creates safety and builds trust. Many of our loving leaders spoke of being the beneficiaries of leaders who provided support for them to take risks or to reach beyond their comfort zones. They spoke of learning from their failures and providing opportunities for their protégées to learn from their own failures without fear that they'd be "dropped" by their mentors if things went wrong. They spoke of feeling confident, and they spoke of wanting to provide a culture in which the people in their organizations who were focused on doing what was right for patients and families would feel confident as well. These are all intentions and actions that create holding.

Holding builds trust. It's what allowed many of the loving leaders we spoke with to feel secure in following their ambitions.

Michael Weahkee spoke about his mentor creating challenging opportunities for him to grow and develop his skills but always within a web of emotional and professional safety. In his words:

> He opened doors for me, but it was up to me to walk through them. I felt safe and confident. I trusted him and his belief in me. Even if I tried and failed, I knew it would be OK. I would be able to learn and do better the next time. There would be no shame.

Holding creates the kind of professional safety he's talking about and gives leaders and potential leaders the confidence to stretch and grow. It removes the fear that a person's failures could get him exiled, which makes space for continuous learning, improvement, and creativity. Holding builds trust. It's what allowed many of the loving leaders we spoke with to feel secure in following their ambitions.

Co-authoring a New Cultural Narrative

As we researched leadership for this chapter, we happened upon this quote: "While it is clear millennials don't really need a lot of trophies, they nevertheless do need a lot of love" (Crowley, 2016). Before any of your current ideas about millennials come rushing to mind, we hope you'll consider that the need for love doesn't make millennials unique. What makes them unique is that they're able to articulate their need for it. Generations X, Y, and Z need love, too. The two baby boomers writing this chapter need love, and so does everyone else.

The workplace is always changing. As we continue to make our way into an age that is alternately called the digital age, the information age, the post-information age, the computer age, the new media age, and (our favorite) the age of relationships, the one thing that's certain is that work and people will continue to change and at a rate that will continue to be nothing short of dizzying. One of the tasks that falls to this and every generation of leaders is to help design the cultural narrative. What stories will we tell about who we are and what matters to us as we move into this new age?

The experience of speaking with these loving leaders provided us with a window into their cultural narratives. They spoke openly about connection, caring, and commitment. Their passion for leading was evident in their expressions and body language. Their openness, authenticity, vulnerability, humility, and commitment to a greater good were easy to see and clearly articulated. They are living a story of connection and caring, nurturing and loving their teams right along with those they serve, and they and others are telling that story as they live it. "Love is a practice," says bell hooks [sic] (2000, p. 165).

We found ourselves greatly humbled by the experience of talking with these eight leaders, and from our brief time with them, we ourselves are inspired to love more, to take more risks, to provide others with the opportunities to take risks, to be more vulnerable, and to fearlessly use the word *love* as we make our way through the world. Imagine working in a culture in which it's normal for people to express love for one another. Imagine receiving care in such a place.

Summary of Key Thoughts

- The presence of love, at all levels of the organization, is a driving force in achieving quality, safety, and exemplary patient-centered experiences.

- It is an act of loving leadership to see something of value in those you serve and to let the person know you see it. Every leader we spoke with talked about someone having seen something in them that they hadn't seen in themselves.

- There is no downside to developing the next generation. If their accomplishments eventually surpass your own, that is cause for celebration.

- Vulnerability and authenticity are no longer seen as liabilities in leaders. Even people in high-powered positions can succeed by truly being who they are rather than projecting a false sense of hypercompetence.

- Loving leaders have a sense that their responsibility for their team's wellbeing extends beyond the walls of the organization. They know that what happens on somebody's 12-hour shift is a small fraction of that person's whole life.

- Loving leaders have the humility to learn from their mistakes, be vulnerable, and take risks. Because humble leaders are more amenable to learning from their mistakes than being crushed by them, humility helps leaders to be more resilient and to model the importance of continuous learning and improvement.

- Loving leaders care about being good examples, good team members, and good people.

- Loving leaders (even those who have no awareness of the four relational practices) find themselves attuning to others simply because they have a genuine interest in the people with whom they share the honor and privilege of working.

- Wondering helps leaders to assume the good intent of the people around them. Further, the culture is markedly improved when leaders visibly spend time wondering with teams or the entire organization.

- The practice of following optimizes the leader's ability to stay informed while also providing others with the experience of being deeply listened to.

- Holding creates professional safety and gives leaders and potential leaders the confidence to stretch and grow. It removes the fear that a person's failures could get him exiled, which makes space for continuous learning, improvement, and creativity.

Reflection

- Consciously practicing attuning, wondering, following, and holding is the key to optimizing every interaction and therefore every relationship. Given this reality, does that make the use of the four relational practices an ethical obligation for leaders? Why or why not?

- Does the cultural narrative of your organization include the word *love*? If not, in what small way could you introduce the idea that love ultimately defines the work of everyone who works in health care?

- Who models humility and loving leadership in your culture? What specific actions stand out for you?

- As Peter Block said: "The best leaders I've known were the ones who sometimes said, 'I don't know.' Loving leadership honors uncertainty." Reflect on whether your culture values expressions of uncertainty. Is it okay to say, "I don't know?" Why or why not?

The good physician treats the disease; the great physician treats the patient who has the disease.

WILLIAM OSLER

CHAPTER SIX

One Physician's Perspective on the Value of Relationships

DAVID ABELSON, MD

Many years after I completed my residency, someone recommended that I read the novel *The House of God,* by Samuel Shem (1978). It was said to present a raucous and hilarious view of the early years in a young physician's life. Instead of laughing, I wept as I read the book. Because so much of it rang true, it triggered a flood of memories and bottled up grief. I cried for the four-year-old who was crushed by a car when he darted out into the street; I cried for his parents, to whom I had to deliver the unfathomable news; I cried for so many patients who died under my watch; and I cried for myself—the young resident named David who tried so hard to be a good resident and in the process buried his humanity and thirst for connections. I cried for that sleep-deprived David who once, when awakened from his on-call bed in the hospital with a phone call announcing a new admission, hoped the patient would die between the emergency room and the intensive care unit because he would "get credit" for the admission but could turn over and go back to sleep. What happened, I wondered, to the compassionate medical student who valued relationships? My tears felt cleansing as I gained insight into how much of my humanity I had buried during residency.

Like most young medical residents, I lacked mature role models who could help me to process, and thus develop from, the physical and emotional intensity of residency. Instead, peer mentors one year ahead of us served to perpetuate a training culture handed down, without critical assessment of its effect, from one young cohort of residents to the next. The culture, in part because of its sheer intensity, was subtly detached from the human elements of medical practice and did not focus much on self-awareness or self-reflection. This kind of culture can still be found in medical education today, and it comes at a high cost to the wellbeing of physicians (Wear, Aultman, Varley, & Zarconi, 2006). It begs a very important question, too: How do we step back into our full humanity after such an experience?

This kind of culture shaped at least three deep-seated assumptions on my part, which are, in fact, common outcomes of most physician training programs: (1) individual exceptionalism reigns supreme, (2) relationships are not part of the "real work" of medicine, and (3) a physician must never be vulnerable.

Many physicians feel that the culture of the organization is not their responsibility.

Throughout our training, we absorbed these assumptions so thoroughly that most docs will resonate with them immediately, although, fortunately, recent residency programs value relational skills more than was evident in my baby boomer physician training. As a byproduct of these assumptions, many physicians feel that the culture of the organization is not their responsibility. There are numerous problems with these assumptions, and they are all intimately connected.

"Individual Exceptionalism Reigns Supreme: I Am Separate From and Above Others"

The first deep-seated assumption is that a physician's attitude of individual exceptionalism should be cultivated and valued. The message is that it is up to you to be exceptional as an individual physician by collecting knowledge and developing skills and judgment and that your patients' lives (and your career) depend on your being exceptional.

The message is important and promotes excellence, but the shadow side of this thinking is that to be exceptional is to be separate and therefore isolated. Indeed, *exceptional* implies that one is better than others—not exactly a solid foundation for teamwork built on partnership and not exactly a desirable element to add to the chemistry of your organization's culture. Additionally, the message that your patient's life depends on you creates a heavy yoke of responsibility, compounding the sense of burdened isolation.

A culture of individual exceptionalism also breeds an emphasis on physician autonomy. If the patient's life is in my hands, and it is solely up to me, then I'd better have the freedom to do what I think is best. Unfortunately, in any given situation, others in the organization may perceive the physician's need for autonomy as bucking the culture—as undermining any sense that we're all in this together.

The biggest problem with a physician's drive for individual exceptionalism is that it subtly and continually separates the physician from the rest of the team. A surgeon might quite reasonably think, "The team is here to make sure I succeed." Though there is some value in the team making the surgeon successful in the operating room, there is danger in devaluing the unique contributions of other team members. It also undermines the kind of commitment that happens when the entire team is focused on the *shared* noble cause of exceptional care and service to the patient. Teamwork is a prerequisite for excellence, and one person thinking of herself as exceptional is not part of the formula for excellent teamwork or ideal outcomes.

I applied what I learned from my physician training to leadership. I was essentially trying to lead as an individual performer. Later, in my role as mentor to developing leaders, I observed that physician leaders needed to traverse a developmental milestone and shift from seeing the job of the team as making them more successful, to seeing their job as making the team more successful.

Individual exceptionalism and its corollary of physician autonomy tend to distance physicians from other team members, leading to the conclusion that organizational culture is not the

> *I observed that physician leaders needed to traverse a developmental milestone and shift from seeing the job of the team as making them more successful, to seeing their job as making the team more successful.*

responsibility of physicians. Of course, culture cannot be escaped; the view that physicians stand outside of the culture actually becomes a destructive assumption within the culture.

"Relationships Are Not Part of the Real Work of Medicine"

There has been a working assumption that relationships are somehow separate from the "real" work of medicine—the real work being the cognitive/technical aspects of diagnosis and treatment. For those with this perspective, healthy relationships are nice but not essential. We hear evidence of the widespread acceptance of this assumption in the common statement: "I know Dr. A is a total jerk, but he is a good doc."

Language in physician training tends to turn patients into objects—problems to be "worked up" and solved—thus casually diminishing patients and undermining the potential for human-to-human connectivity. I vividly recall instructions during an early clinical hospital rotation. "David, go work up the 'lunger' in room 208." The "lunger," a 38-year-old father of three small children, was dying from chronic obstructive pulmonary disease associated with hereditary alpha 1 antitrypsin deficiency. I regret that I let the word "lunger" distance me from this man's anguish and courage in his human struggle.

We worked up "appys," hip fractures, diabetics, acute bellies, and numerous other "conditions." Naming people by their clinical states, we routinely condensed and ignored life experiences, consistently insulating ourselves from the meaning the circumstances have in the lives of our patients.

We do have a choice, of course, in how we talk about things. Imagine replacing the standard clinical term *work up* with a request to *learn about* the person in room 208, who is short of breath with end stage chronic pulmonary disease. Or ceasing to refer to a patient as "the diabetic," which reduces a human being to a condition, and instead saying, "Mrs. Allen with diabetes," which makes clear that Mrs. Allen is a person, and that it's the person, not the disease, who is to be the focus of our care.

The separation of relationships from the real work of medicine can also be seen in differing attitudes toward continuously improving skills. Residency trains physicians in cognitive and technical skills. Understanding that the technical aspects of medicine always advance, we were taught that we needed to work at our technical/cognitive competencies continuously. Traditionally, most residencies have not approached relationship skills as something that must be learned and continuously honed; in fact, they don't even treat the creation and nurturance of therapeutic relationships as a knowledge-based skill. As a result, a subtle but unmistakable message is sent: Physicians do not need to continuously practice and improve their relational skills. This is a tragic and wholly unnecessary oversight. There is a body of knowledge about human response to suffering, and by not making it part of physician education, we reinforce the notion of the body as machine. In the absence of continued learning about the relational aspects of care, physicians are tacitly offered a reprieve from the responsibility to understand the patient's narrative as part of the work of medicine.

> *Physicians are tacitly offered a reprieve from the responsibility to understand the patient's narrative as part of the work of medicine.*

Seeing the cultivation of relationships as not identical to the real work of medicine carries a price. Patients suffer when we are not fully present with them—one human being supporting the healing of another human being. And *we* suffer when we separate ourselves from our own emotions and deny ourselves the renewing energy that comes from human connection. When we separate ourselves from the human pathos around us, we miss opportunities to heal our own wounds by bearing witness to examples of the grace and courage of patients and co-workers dealing with difficulties in their lives. The price of our failure to see relationships as part of the real work of medicine is that we, again, become isolated.

"I Must Never Be Vulnerable"

The third assumption is that we can separate our own human condition from the human condition of patients and co-workers. Medical education, through language and modeling, clearly implies that emotional objectivity and toughness are highly desired qualities.

A study in the Archives of Internal Medicine (Granek, Tozer, Mazzotta, Ramjaun, & Krzyzanowska, 2012) showed that grief is common in medical practice. The study tracked 20 oncologists for nine months to determine if they felt grief when a patient died and how they coped with the grief. In a *New York Times* article about the study, the lead researcher, Leeat Granek, writes:

> ...not only do doctors experience grief, but the professional taboo on the emotion also has negative consequences for the doctors themselves ... More than half of our participants reported feelings of failure, self-doubt, sadness and powerlessness as part of their grief experience, and a third talked about feelings of guilt, loss of sleep and crying. (Granek, 2012)

The study reports:

> The theme of balancing emotional boundaries captured the tension between growing close enough to care about the patients but remaining distant enough to avoid the pain of the loss when the patient died ... [P]atient loss was a unique affective experience that had a smoke-like quality. Like smoke, this grief was intangible and invisible. Nonetheless, it was pervasive, sticking to the physicians' clothes when they went home after work and slipping under the doors between patient rooms. (Granek et al., 2012)

The expectation that we physicians would be hardened and invulnerable didn't take the smoke-like quality of grief into account: You will be overwhelmed and ineffective if you open to the suffering around you. Instead, bury the feelings. Do not acknowledge that ultimately you and everyone you love will someday be a patient. It's as if we were being asked to keep a veil over our shared human wound—the inescapable truth that uncertainty, change, loss, and death are inevitable as we navigate life.

With Great Power Comes Great Responsibility

Ben Parker, uncle of Peter Parker (Spiderman), told a young Spidey, "With great power comes great responsibility." This wisdom summarizes the unique opportunity of physicians to participate in and shape culture instead of pretending to stand outside of it.

As a physician, before embracing the opportunity to consciously contribute to the culture I was part of, I needed to examine how the message from my training that relationships are "nice" but separate from the "real work" of medicine was affecting me.

Separating relationship from the "real work" of medicine and leaving it to others falsely elevates physicians and devalues the contributions of everyone else. In contrast, believing that the ultimate work of medicine is to provide the conditions necessary for the people in our care to regain a sense of wholeness and harmony implies that people in all roles share equally in the potential to contribute. For example, as a young physician resident, I viewed the role of nursing as executing medical orders. I lacked the perspective to value independent nursing diagnoses and interventions related to responses to illness and promoting healing environments that contribute to patient outcomes. I did not have the life experience to appreciate how compassionate human presence—attuning to an individual—supported healing. I failed to fully value nurses as partners whose part in keeping the patient safe was continuously assessing, monitoring, and preventing complications. I held onto full responsibility instead of sharing it, not admitting to myself that it *was* shared. This shared responsibility wouldn't have been a 50/50 split, though; it would have been a true partnership, with each party taking 100% responsibility for his role and trusting his partners to do the same.

I failed to fully value nurses as partners whose part in keeping the patient safe was continuously assessing, monitoring, and preventing complications.

Recognize (Like It or Not) How You Influence Your Team

The de facto leadership position of physicians provides a special opportunity to impact, positively or negatively, the level of interpersonal trust and partnership within teams. Amplification of interpersonal influence through role position provides the power from which flows the responsibility. As a physician—and particularly, later in my career, as a chief medical officer—I discovered the hard way that position amplifies influence and that this included negative influence. As I took on increasing leadership roles, I did not initially appreciate that though I felt like the same person inside, others saw me differently and attached added weight to my words, gestures, and body language. From this new perspective, I looked back at when I was "just another doc." It was only then that I realized that all of my previous sneers and eye-rolls had done lots of damage! And that my vulnerability and authenticity had done a lot of good.

One could argue that it's just plain wrong that role position magnifies personal influence. After all, one human being should not have more influence on interpersonal trust and team dynamics than another human being simply by virtue of role. Paradoxically, in the real world of role influence, physicians can use role to help cultivate a team in which everyone feels equally valued as human beings. Seemingly small gestures, when amplified by role, make a big difference on team dynamics (Yukl, 2013). Simple acts like pitching in to help transfer a patient signal that you value partnership. You are also opening the door to a stronger connection with the team, patient, and family, all of whom are watching. Perhaps even more importantly, when you display humility and vulnerability by asking for a team member's perspective on a patient, asking for help, acknowledging imperfections, and admitting your own mistakes, you create interpersonal trust and safety that are critical for high-functioning teams.

To enhance trust and partnership on teams, physicians need to start by embracing the idea that role amplifies influence. They must also remember that with the power of amplified role influence comes great responsibility. It is deliberate that this chapter follows the chapter, "Loving Leaders Advance Healing Cultures." Physicians must model vulnerability and demonstrate visibly that they value—even love—the human beings with whom they work. Complex health care is highly interdependent, and each person's contribution is vital to extraordinary results. Effective leaders recognize this truth and do their best to demonstrate it in every action and interaction.

Pause for the Patient (An Excellent Use of Power)

A vascular surgeon and good friend uses his role in the operating room (OR) to influence the team. Jeff feels great reverence for the meaning of his work with patients and families but sensed that fellow team members who spent their time dealing only with asleep, draped patients in the OR did not have the same opportunity to connect with meaning. Jeff instituted a "pause for the patient" linked to the often used "pause for the cause." Pause for the cause, implemented to reduce errors in the OR, brings the entire team together immediately before the initial incision to make certain that the right patient is having the right surgery on the right (correct) side with the right equipment. During the pause for the patient, Jeff describes what the surgery means to the patient (which, of course, requires him to take time to *learn* what the surgery means to the patient). For example, Jeff described to the assembled team that the draped patient was a 60-year-old woman diagnosed two months ago with metastatic colon cancer who suddenly developed an embolus (clot) to an artery in her foot; on this day, they were removing the clot. Jeff emphasized to the team how much the woman's life changed in a mere two months. The surgery itself could be thought of as a technical exercise, but in tying it to the bigger picture of the woman's life, he ensured that no one was thinking they were operating on a foot; this was about a person. Knowing Jeff, his reverence was visible, thus signaling vulnerability and enhancing interpersonal trust. At the same time, he made space for team members to deepen their connection with the meaning and impact of their work.

A Call to Action for Physicians: Cultivate Relationships with the People around You

As you know, this book posits three relationship domains: relationship with self, relationship with team members, and relationship with patients and families. You also know that cultivating healthy relationships entails

four relational practices—attuning, wondering, following, and holding—which, in the same way as clinical skills, require constant practice.
Clearly, it makes sense for the call to action in this chapter to be one that
asks physicians (and everyone else) to learn all they can about attuning,
wondering, following, and holding and then to practice these skills as
often as possible in all of their relationships. So do that.

But what I really want to focus on in this call to action is *why*. I want
to focus on the idea that when physicians attune, wonder, follow, and
hold, *they* benefit just as much as anybody else does. Why is that so?

The remarkable side effect to attuning to other people is that you get
to experience attunement yourself, or, as Koloroutis and Trout reminded
us in Chapter Three, you get to experience human connection. Even if
the person you're attuning to cannot or will not attune in return, you still
get to experience the joy of bringing your full self into the act of connecting with another human being. This practice has the immediate effect of
mitigating everything that makes physicians feel separate. Attuning puts
people eye to eye as equals, perhaps softening a physician's need to perpetuate his individual exceptionalism. Attuning is an act of vulnerability,
and the more you do it, the safer you'll feel with your own vulnerability. Finally, attuning changes the culture. Remember the fractal nature
of organizational change: If one part of something changes, the whole is
changed. Therefore, if you attune to anyone, even once, your organization as a whole will be a little more attuned.

There is much to be gained, also, by mindfully experimenting with
the relational practices of wondering and following. To practice wondering, the next time a person in your environment says something to you
or to someone else, just pause and reflect before you speak. If it's socially
appropriate to stay silent, silently wonder about the person without
indulging in any conclusions. Just recognize that there are more things
you don't know about the person (even if you think you know the person
well) than could fill three books. If the circumstance allows it, ask a question that demonstrates following. Be interested in what the person said
or how she looked saying it and ask about it. Stay attuned and see where
the connection goes. The key to the relational practice of following is to
pay attention to the information you're getting from the person you're
attuning to and then to wonder about it. Do your best to keep from *telling*

the person something rather than simply staying open to taking in more information, either through observation or asking questions.

The rewards of wondering and following are a lot like the rewards of attuning. They grow your experience of human connection. You get to experience being a fully connected member of the human family.

Why Holding Is an Essential Practice for Physicians

If you provide someone with a sense of holding—if you make yourself a safe haven—you will add more holding to the culture as a whole. This matters not only because patients and families and your team members need holding to feel safe, secure, creative, and courageous, but because you need it too.

You might even need holding more than many of the people around you. As a physician, you carry something that perhaps no one else in your organization carries. Your fears and worries are as unique within your organization as your responsibilities are. No one else carries exactly what you carry, and it cannot be otherwise. The question is, even though no one can carry it for you, will you allow the rest of the people in the organization to be more meaningfully connected with you as you carry it? Remember, when you put more holding into the world, you put more holding into *your* world.

When you put more holding into the world, you put more holding into your world.

The very nature of our work calls to the forefront the impermanence of our own lives and our desires to keep ourselves and our loved ones safe. It reveals the universal human wound of dealing with the fragility of life as we face the truth that we, like all other human beings, are doing the best we can to make sense of the complex processes of birth, aging, illness, injury, trauma, and death. Why would any of us choose to be alone on a journey as hard as this one?

The messages of our training have set physicians up to feel separate, isolated, and alone, but these messages need not dictate our professional ways of being. If we want to feel connected, it is incumbent upon us to connect. If we want to feel held, it is incumbent upon us to hold others and to allow them to hold us when holding is offered. Intentionally holding others will not just be "one more thing to do." It will be the thing you do that makes all of the other things you do easier. You *are* connected. You're connected to your team, to your patients and families, and to your organization. Acknowledging that inherent connection takes less energy than it takes to fight it. And while no one else can carry for you the things that you alone must carry, every burden is lighter for those of us who are committed to forging and nurturing healthy relationships.

Summary of Key Thoughts

- Common unintended outcomes of physician training programs can include believing that (1) individual exceptionalism reigns supreme, (2) relationships are not part of the real work of medicine, (3) a physician's own sense of vulnerability and mortality are best kept out of the equation altogether, and (4) the culture of the health care organization is not a physician's concern.

- A physician's drive for individual exceptionalism and autonomy subtly and continually separates the physician from the rest of the team while negating the kind of commitment that happens when the entire team is focused on the shared noble cause of exceptional care and service to the patient.

- If physicians don't see relationships as part of the real work of medicine, patients and physicians both suffer because they are cut off from the renewing energy of human connection.

- With great power comes great responsibility. Because a physician's role amplifies interpersonal influence, physicians are responsible for cultivating healthy team relationships.

- Complex health care is highly interdependent, and each person's contribution is vital to extraordinary results. Effective physicians recognize this truth and do their best to demonstrate it in every action and interaction.

- A fortunate side effect of attuning to other people is that you get to experience attunement yourself; you get to experience human connection.

- The relational practices of wondering and following help you experience being a fully connected member of the human family.

- Physicians benefit from holding others, partly because it creates more holding for themselves as well. Holding helps people feel safe, secure, creative, and courageous—all things that every last one of us could use more of.

Reflection

- No matter what your role is, reflect on the mindsets and assumptions you carry as a result of your professional education.

- Consider the following: "With great power comes great responsibility." In what ways do you exercise your own power to shape the culture?

- The surgeon who called for a "pause for the patient" influenced his team to attune to and wonder about the *person* on the table and to connect with the meaning and purpose of their work. What conversation, process, or structure could your team create that would help everyone stay mindful of the humanity of every person every time?

- If you are a physician, what are some ways that you might allow yourself to be held by the rest of the team? If you are not a physician, what are some ways you might hold your physician colleagues?

In a clinical setting, authentic human connection cannot be mandated. It can, however, be a clearly articulated expectation, a shared purpose, a goal, and a standard.

Mary Koloroutis and Michael Trout

CHAPTER SEVEN

Embedding Relational Competence

KRISTEN LOMBARD, DONNA WRIGHT, AND TARA NICHOLS

Health care executives across the nation identify the patient and family experience as one of their top priorities. While leaders agree that a positive patient experience is essential to quality care, many organizations struggle with how to bring a consistently positive patient experience to life in their culture. A variety of customer service strategies and tactics have not yielded the desired results (Wolf, 2013). While customer service strategies have led to a tangible shift in hospitality and responsiveness in health care settings, they have not achieved the more substantial impact of helping clinicians and support staff members to connect with patients and their loved ones with compassion and a healing therapeutic focus.

Additionally, due partly to the breakneck pace of technical innovation in health care, there has been an overemphasis on the tasks of caregiving at the expense of developing and fostering the relational competence that must necessarily accompany them. In reality, any task that includes a person is inseparable from the relational aspects of care; these tasks actually *require* relational competence if they are to be performed effectively. As the movement to strengthen the patient experience evolves, there is greater understanding that "just as it would not be thought acceptable for clinicians to lack technical proficiency,

> *Just as it would not be thought acceptable for clinicians to lack technical proficiency, it cannot be deemed acceptable for clinicians to lack relational proficiency.*

it cannot be deemed acceptable for clinicians to lack relational proficiency" (Koloroutis & Trout, 2012, p. 28).

There is also, in recent years, greater understanding that if relational competence is to become embedded within any organization, it must be expected, developed, nurtured, practiced, reinforced, and evaluated. Cultivating relational competence aligns with all patient-centered missions, visions, and values; relational competence can and must become a cultural way of being.

If relational competence is to become embedded within any organization, it must be expected, developed, nurtured, practiced, reinforced, and evaluated.

The purpose of this chapter is to provide leaders and clinicians with a competency-based framework for individual development and organizational enculturation of the four therapeutic practices of attuning, wondering, following, and holding. This chapter includes a brief review of the practices with an emphasis on the behaviors that actualize them, the importance of understanding the knowledge base behind them, the mindset necessary for the practices to become embodied by clinicians, and what care looks like when the therapeutic practices support the "therapeutic use of self."

Bringing the Therapeutic Practices to Life

Patients and families are asking for clinicians to make a genuine human connection with them. Figure 7.1 provides definitions of the therapeutic practices of attuning, wondering, following, and holding; below each practice is a list of core competencies that facilitate a genuine human connection. The purpose of identifying core competencies for each therapeutic practice is to support clinicians and leaders in embedding the practices into their care settings through a competency development and assessment process.

Attuning
The practice of being present in the moment and tuning in to an individual or situation.

Connects with the patient and family with a focus on their state of being (physical, emotional, mental, and spiritual).

Notices verbal and nonverbal cues indicating anxiety or distress and responds appropriately.

Tunes in to the energy in the room, including one's own energy, proximity, and pace of communication.

Communicates acceptance and respect for the person receiving care through listening, spoken words, and body language.

Gives focused attention to the person and minimizes interruptions to care.

Recognizes the potential for the EHR and other technical processes to interfere with the therapeutic connection, and takes appropriate action to stay tuned in to the person.

Conveys openness, transparency, and interest in the person.

Conveys a sturdy, compassionate, and nonjudgmental presence.

Wondering
The practice of being genuinely interested in a person. It requires an open-hearted curiosity about what can be learned about this unique individual, while intentionally suspending assumptions and judgment.

Conveys genuine interest in the person receiving care.

Asks open-ended questions.

Suspends own agenda as appropriate and seeks to learn about the person.

Communicates an openness and desire to listen and learn from the patient and family.

Conveys respect for human diversity, patient and family history, and culture.

Avoids assumptions and consciously suspends judgments; is aware of potential for personal bias and refrains from labeling.

Stays open and curious to new data and information about the person.

Remembers that everyone has a unique backstory that will affect their interactions and responses to care.

Challenges oneself and one's own mindset to reflect the complete situation and experience of all involved.

Following

The practice of listening to and focusing on what an individual is teaching us about what matters most to her or him and allowing that information to guide our interactions. It requires consciously suspending our own agenda.

Collaborates with the patient and family as involved partners in their own care.

Listens with a focus on what matters most to the person.

Provides sufficient time and attention for the patient and family to share what is on their minds.

Refrains from interrupting, correcting, or rushing to fix things before hearing the person's perspective.

Provides care that is consistent with what the patient and family say matters to them.

Notices and responds to the person's cues and/or expressed preferences re: proximity, eye contact, touch, preferred name, etc.

Listens to and validates the person with empathetic sounds and conscious body language.

Clarifies and seeks to resolve areas of concern and/or disagreement.

Builds a sense of safety and trust by remembering specific patient and family needs and requests.

Holding

The practice of intentionally creating a safe haven to protect the safety and dignity of an individual.

Conveys a fundamental regard for the dignity and privacy of all persons needing care.

Acts with integrity and care by following through on all commitments.

Asks for help when necessary to meet patient and family needs.

Communicates information about the patient and family to the rest of the health care team in respectful terms and language.

Avoids derogatory labels or descriptors that may bias team members and interfere with ability to remain open and therapeutic.

Shares information and proactively attends to transitions so that the patient and family know what is happening and what to expect in their care.

Participates in and encourages consistent and visible teamwork to safeguard the wellbeing of the patient and family.

Remains a steady presence even in the face of strong emotions and crisis.

Recognizes anger as an expression of fear and distress and takes action to alleviate distress.

Figure: 7.1: See Me as a Person Therapeutic Practices: Core Competencies (Developed by Koloroutis & Trout, 2017.)

This table of relational core competencies applies to the therapeutic care of all patients. However, these competencies can be tailored to support clinicians in caring for specific patient populations. A list of relational core competencies tailored for clinicians working in pain management and comfort care can be found in Appendix A.

What Is a Competency Development and Assessment Process?

The *Oxford English Dictionary* defines *competency* as "the ability to do something successfully or effectively" (2016). The purpose of engaging in a competency development and assessment process is to help a group of people *gain* and *demonstrate* the ability to do something successfully or effectively. As Figure 7.2 shows, a competency consists of a knowledge base, a particular mindset (i.e., a way of thinking), and specific behaviors that bring the competency to life.

Defining competencies for technical skills has traditionally been a fairly straightforward endeavor. Technical skills are concrete, observable, measurable, and can be clearly defined. It is much more challenging to define, describe, teach, and measure relational success and effectiveness. Since relational practices have historically been perceived as difficult to measure, they have often been left out of the competency process altogether. While clinicians understand the importance of remaining current and continuously honing their technical competence, relational competence has not been viewed in the same way.

Why Knowledge and Mindset Must Accompany Application

Relational competence develops over time and requires intellectual, emotional, and professional maturation. In order to demonstrate consistent relational competence, clinicians need to understand the knowledge base and the mindset that underpin the therapeutic practices. It is through knowledge and understanding that we begin to embody the practices. To be fully competent in anything requires that we understand the "why"—the theory, research, experience, values, and ethics—behind the application of the desired behaviors. (See Figure 7.2.)

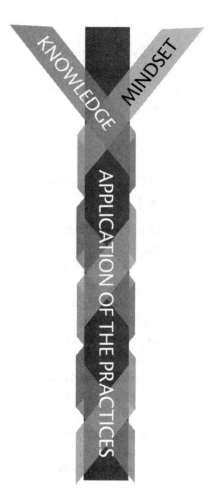

The *See Me as a Person* book and workshop provide the knowledge base and help cultivate the mindset conducive to the consistent application of the practices of attuning, wondering, following, and holding. The knowledge base underpinning the therapeutic practices includes understanding the human response to illness and crisis, the neuroscience of attunement and mindfulness, the ethical and moral principles guiding human caring, and the therapeutic use of self. The mindset necessary for the cultivation of relational competence includes humility, continuous learning, compassion for self and others, and healthy teamwork. As people begin to understand the knowledge base, their mindsets begin to shift as they assimilate what they've learned.

Figure 7.2: Knowledge, Mindset, and Application

Studying and reflecting on the knowledge base and mindset underlying the four relational practices is necessary if the behavior change is to be sustainable. Consider this core competency for the practice of *holding* from Figure 7.1: "Provides care that is consistent with what the patient and family say matters to them." This important competency may be forgotten or neglected unless it is aligned with the clinician's beliefs, values, and thinking. The learning outcome will become memorable when the clinician connects to the knowledge-based understanding, such as knowing that a common human response to illness is to feel vulnerable and powerless, and that patients feel safer when clinicians attune and demonstrate active listening. A competency process that tells people what to do but not *why* will fall short.

> *By clearly defining what constitutes relational competence in a work area, we make relational competence accessible, teachable, and measurable.*

By clearly defining what constitutes relational competence in a work area, we make relational competence accessible, teachable, and measurable. Only then does it become reasonable that relational competence is an articulated performance expectation.

Awareness of Our Mindset

The mindset—or *way of thinking*—that is most conducive to sustained application of the practices includes commitment to the following:

- One's own growth and learning

- Teamwork and colleagueship

- Compassion for self and others

- Humility and genuine interest in learning about each unique person

The following example demonstrates what can happen when a leader chooses to make her way of thinking visible and engages the team to learn with her and improve patient care.

Reflection: Modeling Self-Awareness to Counteract Bias

Dr. Green entered our pre-rounding meeting and placed the rounding list of patients on a table where it was easily seen. "Did you see who is back again?! Mr. Jones! That patient drives me crazy!" She discussed this patient for a full minute with disdain; then she stopped talking. The quiet in the room was deafening. Everyone was wondering who would speak first. After a few moments, Dr. Green said, as a palpable sense of humility washed over her, "Why did I do that? Coming into rounds talking about a patient in this manner"? We didn't know how to respond. Her earlier outburst was completely out of character for Dr. Green; after all, it was she who had initiated a caring and holistic approach to pain management.

Dr. Green continued, "We must always be willing to examine how our biases impact our patient care." She went on to discuss the beliefs and assumptions behind why she felt as she did and explained that without self-examination her beliefs and assumptions about the patient could drive the way she interacted with the patient, leading to less than optimal care. Dr. Green continued, "We are going to review our differential diagnosis for this patient to make sure we are providing the very best care. When we round today I ask that you all hold me accountable. I need to go in, sit down with this patient, and listen to what he needs." Someone asked, "Don't we do this for all patients?" Dr. Green replied, "We should, and in this situation, I know I have a bias against this patient; I cannot allow that to interfere with how I treat him. My efforts need to be even more intentional, and I'm asking the team to help me."

This reflection teaches the power of recognizing our mindset, examining our own beliefs, and considering their effect on patient care. Dr. Green, an experienced practitioner of medicine, demonstrated a willingness to learn and grow, making herself the example, saying out loud what many were thinking. As a leader, she engaged the team in reflecting on how disrespectful thoughts could impact patient care. She challenged her own assumptions, opened her heart, and asked for support. By making her internal process visible to the team, Dr. Green influenced the awareness and thinking of her team members about how their beliefs could impact their behavior. As a leader, Dr. Green raised the potential for such self-examination to become a cultural norm.

Using Competency Assessment to Embed Relational Competence into Practice

Leaders will be successful in embedding relational competence when they cultivate a shared vision and articulate expectations for relational competence. They must also understand what it takes to promote and support professional development. In the competency assessment pathway in Figure 7.3, three levels of competence are defined as (1) gaining knowledge of the practices, (2) visible commitment to an open mindset, and (3) consistent application of the practices.

A three-level competency process defines a pathway that sets the minimum expectation required to be demonstrated at each level (Wright, 2005, 2015). In this journey to relational competence, individuals grow as they progress in applying the therapeutic practices.

LEVEL 3
Consistently attune, wonder, follow, and hold; integrate reflection into daily behaviors and relationships.

LEVEL 2
Commit to an open mindset, desire to learn, and reflection. Adopt mindset to improve relational competence and apply the practices.

LEVEL 1
Gain knowledge of attuning, wondering, following, and holding as therapeutic practices; begin to use the terminology; explore and reflect on the related knowledge base.

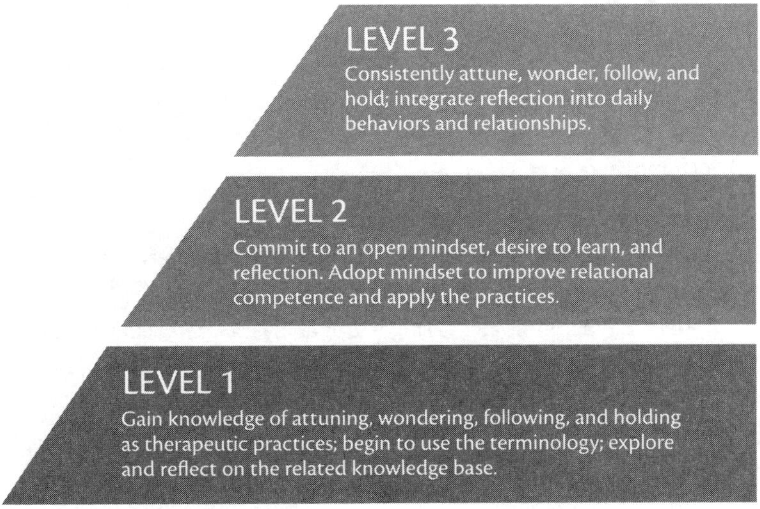

Figure 7.3: The Developmental Pathway to Relational Competence

With the goal of advancing a relationship-based culture, the three-level competency process helps to create an environment in which the four therapeutic practices are not just understood but are, over time, consistently embodied.

In this three-level competency process, **competency statements** guide the learning and application of the practices. **Competency verification methods** are ways to evaluate whether a competency has been met. What follows in Figure 7.4 is a selection of sample competency statements and verification methods for each level in the pathway to relational competence.

Level 1: Gain Knowledge of the Practices

Competency statements for Level 1

- The clinician demonstrates awareness of related knowledge base; can name and define the four therapeutic practices.
- The clinician demonstrates attuning by taking in and observing verbal and nonverbal cues and expressions.
- The clinician demonstrates ability to give focused attention to the person and minimize interruptions to care.

Competency Verification Methods for Level 1

- Tests (can be in module format, presentation/class, or dialogue groups)
- Participation in reflection circles
- Exemplar story describing the use and outcomes of the identified competency
- Simulation lab exercises

Level 2: Demonstrate an Open Mindset

Competency statements for Level 2

- The clinician demonstrates awareness of own values, beliefs, strengths, and challenges in various clinical situations.
- The clinician demonstrates willingness to apply the therapeutic practices.
- The clinician shows a commitment and openness to attuning, wondering, following, and holding in daily interactions.
- The clinician integrates therapeutic practice concepts into specific patient populations and situations.

Competency Verification Methods for Level 2

- Participation in reflection circles and discussion groups
- Sharing examples of actual or potential relational situations that were successful or not
- Sharing of practice experiences through case studies
- Exemplar story describing demonstration of an open mindset toward using the practices
- Simulation lab exercises

Level 3: Consistent Application of the Practices

Competency Statements for Level 3

- The clinician consistently demonstrates attuning, wondering, following, and holding in daily interactions with patients and families, team members, and other relationships.
- The clinician demonstrates the ability to maintain a steady presence even in the face of strong emotions and crises.
- The clinician demonstrates consistent ability to reflect on therapeutic practices and collaborative relationships.

Competency Verification Methods for Level 3

- Patient experience feedback
- Patient letters
- Colleague feedback and/or peer review
- Observation (can be done at handoff reports, huddles, case conferences, direct care, etc.)
- Exemplar story about consistent application of the practices
- Simulation lab exercises

Figure 7.4: Sample Competency Statements and Verification Methods

Each clinician's competency pathway may look different, according to the competencies she needs to develop or deepen. While a group may decide to all work on the same competencies, it is ideal for individuals to also identify for themselves practices they will work on in order to develop more deeply and consistently. Clinicians should partner with their formal leaders to identify appropriate verification methods.

The Leader's Role in Embedding the Four Therapeutic Practices in the Culture

Leaders at all levels have the responsibility and accountability for embedding the therapeutic practices into the organization's culture. Most of that responsibility will be met through consistent modeling of the therapeutic practices in every relationship. Attuning, wondering, following, and holding are the how-to for all healthy relationships, so the more they are modeled by leaders, the sooner the relational competencies will become normative. Leaders committing to the relational competencies and engaging in healthy relationships are advancing the transformation of the organization's culture. Without such modeling, nothing else the leader says or does will move the group toward embedding the therapeutic practices in their work. Part of the leader's job is to advance the mission of the organization by inspiring the shared purpose of providing high-quality, safe, and compassionate care to patients and their loved ones. In relationship-based cultures this is achieved through a balance of intentionally designed structures, effective processes, and committed and competent people. A vital part of how leaders exemplify a commitment to the best possible care is modeling relational excellence.

A vital part of how leaders exemplify a commitment to the best possible care is modeling relational excellence.

The competencies in Figure 7.1 are designed for patient situations; however, many of them apply or can easily be adapted to relationships between colleagues and even in our relationships with ourselves. For example, leaders may choose to use a competency such as "Avoids assumptions and consciously suspends judgments; is aware of potential for personal bias and refrains from labeling" as a touchstone for their own or their team's development. (A list of relational core competencies adapted for teams can be found in Appendix B.)

Partner with Staff to Create Systems and Processes That Support Use of the Practices

While there is always something each individual caregiver can do to improve the relational aspects of care, these individual actions will become norms only if the organizational culture is actively focused on identifying barriers and improving structures and processes to support human connection. Consider this everyday example described by a nurse working in an inpatient hospital setting.

Reflection: Constant Interruptions

I was working at a hospital where nurses carried staff cell phones. All the calls from lab, central supply, telemetry, call lights, and anyone who needed to contact the nurse came to the phone. The nurse who was orienting me to the unit was interrupted seven times during a 12-minute conversation as she was attempting to explain a procedure to her patient. After we left the room, I asked, "Why do you answer your phone while you're in the room with the patient? Aren't you concerned that it's interfering with your relationship?" She stated, "If we don't answer our phone, it is tracked, and we get called into the manager's office to explain why we're not answering our phone immediately. It goes on our performance record, and I need my job! It's just easier to stop what we're doing and answer the phone." I thought, "Is anyone tracking how all of these interruptions affect quality, safety, and the patient's experience of care?"

When examples of processes that impede relationships come to light, it's up to leaders to actively partner with staff members to identify strategies to overcome barriers and redesign systems to support human connection. As this everyday example brings to life, there can be an insidious tolerance of systems that directly interfere with human connection. It takes strong leader-staff partnerships to find new ways to resolve long-standing problems.

Develop (or Release) Staff Members Who Do Not Come Along

Emphasizing the importance of the relational competencies with people who are ready and eager to engage is a great starting point and is energizing for all involved. It is equally important, however, for leaders to address those team members who are ignoring the expectation for developing relational competence, attempting to disrupt the changes through resistive behavior, and/or criticizing or even intimidating those who embrace the change.

Consider this example of a team member who is actively resisting a cultural change:

Reflection: A Potential Threat to the Culture

One member of the team has a pattern of being verbally disrespectful to other team members. Other team members use their new relational practices and step forward with courage to openly discuss a current incident, using attuning, wondering, following, and holding. Still, the person's behavior does not change. The verbally disrespectful team member escalates the behaviors or isolates himself from the rest of the team, making it almost impossible for the team to collaborate effectively. Team members ask for leadership support in this troubled situation, but no action is taken. The person's behavior is thus tolerated, and the initiative to improve relational competence in the organization is sabotaged. People begin to say, "Why bother doing this anymore? Nobody else seems to care."

In this example, team members brought a difficult issue forward, but there was no follow-through by the leader, and no corrective action was initiated. When leaders follow through with expectations by actively coaching and mentoring, and yet the behavior doesn't change, a disciplinary process is necessary. The leader's role is to demonstrate that all team members are held to the same standards and expectations. These actions are critical to embedding the cultural change and cultivating psychological safety within the team.

The Silent Treatment Study (Maxfield, Grenny, Lavandero, & Groah, 2010) reminds us that when caregivers avoid communication with colleagues or work around colleagues with aberrant behavior, there is a risk of significant harm to patients and a compromise to a healthy work environment. In this study of 6,500 caregivers, 58% indicated that they either felt unsafe to speak up about an issue or were unable to get others to address the issue. In our fieldwork, we see and hear that incidents of this sort are still impacting health care teams.

If the goal is to embed the four therapeutic practices within a unit, department, or organization, it must become an expectation that *everyone's* performance will be evaluated on their relational competence, not just the people who choose to engage. Leaders seldom find the movement of an employee out of a department or organization pleasant, but it is an action that must be taken when it is being done to safeguard the best possible teamwork and patient care and to continuously strengthen and advance the culture within which care is provided.

How We Know We've Reached Our Goal: The Therapeutic Use of Self

The therapeutic use of self means bringing all of who you are to an interaction. It has been defined as "the ability to use theory, experiential knowledge, and self-awareness, and to explore one's impact on others" ("Therapeutic use of self," 2003). Therapeutic use of self has been taught and advocated in several professional disciplines; an early reference in family therapy literature is *The Use of Self in Therapy* (Baldwin & Satir, 1987); occupational therapy scholar Mosey (1986) proposed the conscious use of

> *The therapeutic use of self means bringing all of who you are to an interaction.*

self as a therapeutic tool. Wosket (1999) applied the concept to individual counseling practice and outcomes. Nursing theorists have emphasized therapeutic relationships (Peplau, 1991) and authentic presence (Watson, 2008). A current leading scholar and proponent of the therapeutic use of self is Renee R. Taylor, author of *The Intentional Relationship: Occupational Therapy and Use of Self* (2008).

Reflection: Therapeutic Use of Self (a.k.a. Application of Attuning, Wondering, Following, and Holding)

Tara was caring for Helen, a patient who was short of breath. Helen's condition had improved, but she was still on oxygen and had several intravenous medications infusing. All of these therapies and her physical state made it difficult and unsafe for her to walk to the bathroom. Tara could see in the patient's eyes that she did not want to use a bedpan. Helen asked, "Can I get up?" Tara helped her to the bedside commode, and Helen asked for toilet paper to clean herself. Tara said, "I need to stay with you to keep you safe, and I need to be the one to clean you to help conserve the oxygen you use." Helen started to cry. Tara told Helen that she was honored to care for her and that her commitment to Helen's safety included caring for her skin so that she would not get bedsores. When Tara was done, she gave Helen a warm wash cloth to wash her hands and then washed her own hands. Helen asked her to come closer. She took Tara's hands in hers and kissed them. She told Tara she was an angel—that all the time she had been in the hospital no one recognized how important it was for her to get up, or made her feel safe to get up, and so she had been cleaning herself, despite being weak and short of breath. She concluded that Tara cared for her with compassion and grace. Tara felt that by being fully present and attuned, wondering out loud about what Helen needed, following where she was spiritually and physically, and designing her care around what she learned from those actions, she held Helen in dignity and provided safe and comprehensive care. Being who she was as an individual, and also drawing on her scientific knowledge, Tara demonstrated the four therapeutic practices that embody the therapeutic use of self.

We are called to transform our organizations into cultures in which people come together in relational unity to promote individual healing, while advancing systems, processes, and environments that strengthen therapeutic and collegial relationships. Practically, we have demystified the therapeutic relationship and described a framework for clinicians to develop relational practices, to take ownership within the caregiving experience, and to engage themselves fully in their professional work.

Summary of Key Thoughts

- Relational competence is essential for patient and family comfort and must be provided along with our technological expertise.

- Knowledge, mindset, and application are inexorably intertwined; knowledge and mindset make possible the consistent application of the therapeutic practices.

- The three-level competency process builds on a specific knowledge base and on helping individuals develop a mindset that is conducive to the attuned application of the practices.

- Each clinician's competency pathway may look different, according to what skills he or she is needing to develop or deepen.

- Leadership has a role in embedding the four therapeutic practices. Leaders must follow through with the expectation that all employees interact with a basic level of relational competence; leaders must also model the practices, help create systems and processes to support them, and develop or terminate staff who are resistant to coming along.

- Positive interprofessional relationships, as well as positive relationships with patients and their loved ones, rarely just happen; these relationships require the cultivation of safe interpersonal environments in which colleagues can continually practice new ways of interacting therapeutically.

Reflection

- What kinds of outcomes would you anticipate if relational competence became an expectation in your organization? Would efforts be successful? Why or why not?

- How does an expectation of relational competence relate to your organization's mission and values?

- Behaviors are based on belief systems, which can develop surreptitiously over a lifetime. Use the following questions to reflect alone or with a group:

  - What do I believe about the value of authentic relationships at work?

  - In what ways are my beliefs reflected in how I engage with people?

  - Do I believe that each person has something to teach me that is important?

  - What do I believe about the energy I bring to work relationships and how my energy impacts others?

- Learning and practicing relational behaviors engenders vulnerability and risk. How safe would you say the learning environment is in your unit, department, or organization? How might the organization change in order to embrace vulnerability and learning?

It is literally true that you can succeed best and quickest by helping others succeed.

Napoleon Hill

CHAPTER EIGHT

The Role of Human Resources in Advancing Culture

Brett Long, Donna Wright, and Ann Flanagan Petry

Every important health care outcome is achieved through people. It is people who assure safety, provide quality clinical services, create a great patient experience, provide caring and healing environments, and manage financial value. Real value is generated by people working in healthy, productive relationships with other people. Since collaboration and relationships are the foundation of interprofessional team-based care, it shouldn't be surprising that chief executive officers (CEOs) rank recruiting and retaining the best people as their number one challenge. Yet, surprisingly, the department most often responsible for talent management, human resources (HR), is ranked 8th or 9th in functional importance by most CEOs (Ray et al., 2012), which may explain why HR frequently settles into a more transactional role rather than a strategic one.

In this chapter, we will discuss what high-performing HR leaders do to build outstanding teams and accelerate success. Additionally, we will discuss how organizations are recognizing that developing people can't be an afterthought. Forward-thinking organizations are embedding relational competence, starting with skills such as self-awareness and attuning, into every step of the talent life cycle: recruiting, selection, onboarding, individual and team development, succession planning, performance reviews, and even terminations of employment (Bartram, 2007; Collins & Clark, 2003; Kepes & Delery, 2006; Lengnick-Hall, 2010).

Human Resources Leaders and Operational Leaders as Partners

It is the CEO, in strong partnership with the chief human resources officer (CHRO), who is ultimately responsible for hiring and developing people who are congruent with the organization's mission and strategic imperatives. The CEO-CHRO partnership must have a crystal-clear focus on developing culture and the people who create the culture—which is everyone. The quality of this partnership sets the tone for the rest of the organization's people strategies and people processes. The partnership must be healthy, visible, and collegial.

Partnerships at all levels are improved when people are clear about their primary responsibilities. In Appendix C, we offer a simple tool to help facilitate a conversation between operational and HR leaders to maximize clarity and minimize potential areas of misunderstanding about roles and responsibilities. Reviewing and discussing roles and responsibilities can bring clarity and help nurture a genuine partnership between HR professionals and operations managers.

In our experience, a good structural model to catalyze partnerships between HR professionals and operational managers is one that includes the role of a human resources business partner (HRBP) (Mazor, Alburey, Volini, Bowden, & Stephan, 2014; Schatsky & Schwartz, 2015; Vonderhaar, 2016). In this model, HRBPs partner with operational leaders in specific departments and/or service lines and serve as a complete resource for leaders in those areas. The operational leaders, in turn, nurture the partnership by including the HRBPs in appropriate meetings, proactively consulting with them about HR concerns, and inviting them to join the team in celebrations of success. Operational leaders bring the HRBP into their department or service line as a visible and valued partner.

A significant benefit of this model is relationship continuity which allows the HRBP to become a trusted advisor and an objective coach for the leaders of those departments and service lines. People in the HRBP role provide human-centered expertise to leaders to assist with building team effectiveness, help leaders identify and compensate for their own blind spots, and act as strategic partners in facilitating optimal team structures. When a true partnership exists between the operational leader and the HRBP, the HRBP can help elevate the caliber of people and teams. For example, a CNO described the benefits of collaboration with her human resources team: "I count on HR for leading with a shared vision, presence, honesty, a different point of view, appreciation for the understanding that our work touches patients in meaningful ways, keeping us all out of trouble (keeping me out of trouble—the brutal truth), and assistance in celebrating success and spreading the love" (Personal communication, January 25, 2017).

Because of the volume of people who are entering or exiting the organization or experiencing other sorts of changes or challenges, the relationship between HR and operational leaders can be stressful no matter how much interpersonal trust they share. A strong partnership within a collaborative culture helps leaders from both operations and HR to navigate these challenges.

In a relationship-based culture, the HR team can and must be cultural ambassadors, modeling attuning, wondering, following, and holding in every interaction.

As the previous chapter stated, it is the responsibility of every person in the organization to be relationally competent. When HR and operational leaders work together with a clear aim to model and actively embed relational competence, they are uniquely positioned to advance a relationship-based culture. Additionally, the HR team has an amplified opportunity to influence the entire organization because *all* of their work is people- and culture-centered and because they interact with people in every stage of the talent life cycle. In a relationship-based culture, the HR team can and must be cultural ambassadors, modeling attuning, wondering, following, and holding in every interaction.

Recruiting and Selecting Relational Leaders and Team Members

Designing systems and practices that build and sustain a high-performing organization starts at the very beginning of the talent life cycle: recruiting and selecting people who fit the organization's expectations of both technical and relational competence. Our first opportunity to communicate the importance of this balance is often in job postings. This is a critical opportunity to promote the soul of the organization and explicitly describe the profile of the person who will thrive in this environment. A well-articulated job posting sifts out those who don't fit the culture and excites and energizes those who do.

Just as we aim to attract candidates who match our technical and relational values, high-performing organizations align recruiting and hiring practices with their cultural values. Consider the story of a candidate we'll call Jennifer, who interviewed with a large health care system. The initial job-screening process was automated. A recorded voice asked cursory questions. Jennifer talked into a camera, answering the computer prompts. There was no verbal or nonverbal feedback, only a beep for her to continue or stop. The impersonal process left her feeling disheartened. Even if Jennifer is a good fit and is offered a job, what are her first impressions of the organization? What has she perceived about the culture through this impersonal interaction?

A well-articulated job posting sifts out those who don't fit the culture and excites and energizes those who do.

In contrast, take a moment to think about a hiring process you've experienced as a prospective employee. Did you ever have an interview that felt "right"? Afterward, you might have reflected: "We really clicked." If so, chances are you experienced an attuned connection. This attunement flipped a positive switch in you and was likely an influential factor in your decision to take the job. Indeed, in interviewing, nonverbal messages and cues provide great insight into personality as well as organizational culture, and these impressions matter. Notably, when attunement is the norm, HR interviewers model the importance of relational competency. Remember, they are the face of the organization to potential new hires.

Because relational competence is so crucial in health care, there is growing interest in pre-employment assessments to screen job applicants. For example, Talent Plus, Inc. has studied top performers in health care for more than 25 years. They provide a pre-hiring assessment that identifies discrete talents in individual candidates, including relational competence, which is a predictor of performance excellence. This type of assessment offers insight into a person's abilities in attuning, emotional flexibility, curiosity, motivation, and more. Beyond the tool's use for initial screening, meaningful understanding of the assessment results offer managers insight into employees' strengths and interests. Ultimately, assessments of this sort have the potential to fast-track coaching, partnering, and teaming (Rath, 2014; Thompson & Ahrens, 2015).

Additionally, situational and behavioral interviewing methods offer candidates a chance to show an employer behaviors that are differentiating and that uncover relational aptitude. Behavioral interviewing is a process in which the candidate describes personal experiences with challenging situations; situational interviewing asks candidates to describe how they would react to a hypothetical situation. Methods such as these allow us to more completely assess a person's relational competence.

Relationship-Based Onboarding of New Leaders and Team Members

A new employee's first day is an extraordinary opportunity to inspire a shared purpose and a new social contract of common values that will bind people together. Furthermore, the best onboarding practices address two basic outcomes: (1) What will make this person feel welcome? and (2) What will contribute to this person's early and ongoing success? All onboarding activities must help advance these two outcomes, and therefore must provide the new person with all the technical knowledge and all the relational knowledge needed to be successful. For example, it is important to have new team members' agendas for the first day designed to help them feel welcome and cared for (their leader welcoming them at the front door, lunch with someone familiar) as well as functionally important (their system login is activated, they have a computer that works and a preceptor or mentor engaged to support their learning for the first 90 days).

Effective onboarding starts with early planning—right after the decision to hire—and continues for at least 90 days, no matter what the position. A key to successful onboarding is effective partnering between the operational leader and the HR partner. The operational leader has primary responsibility to onboard the new team member and relies heavily on the human resources team and infrastructure to do it effectively. Together, the leader and HR will provide the new employee a well-balanced, practical, and inspirational introduction to the organization and the local team. For those leaders who hire many people, personalizing this process can seem like a monumental undertaking, but with strong HR partnership, the process can be both effective and efficient.

Developing Leaders and Team Members

A strong HR team plays an important role in advising and assisting executives and all leaders in building a culture of continuous individual and team improvement. In high-performing organizations, human resources is a true partner in building healthy, effective teams. This includes developing a culture in which performance expectations are clear, individual and team development are priorities, and future leaders are sought out and developed.

While succession planning generally aims to assess team members' advancement potential or leadership readiness, in a relationship-based culture this process recognizes that candidates must also possess relational competence.

In partnership with top leaders, HR leaders build and manage a relational, transparent, and respectful succession planning process. While succession planning generally aims to assess team members' advancement potential or leadership readiness, in a relationship-based culture this process recognizes that candidates must also possess relational competence. Recall for a moment the loving leaders profiled earlier in this book. It is their relational competence that makes them leaders others are proud and happy to follow.

Transformational HR leaders play an important role in creating the conditions that make trust building, caring, and attuning behaviors easier to develop and actualize. These behaviors will become normative in our organizations only when we directly link our work with our core values and personal visions of our best selves (Bono & Judge, 2003; Boyatzis & McKee, 2005; Piccolo & Colquitt, 2006; Shamir, House, & Arthur, 1993). HR leaders are in a position to choose, design, and/or deliver numerous education opportunities into which they can weave relational knowledge and skill building.

One simple yet effective process for leadership and team development is to incorporate strengths-based development plans that can be customized to fit the needs of the people involved. People are invited to explore what gives them meaning and purpose in their work, identify their top strengths, determine concrete ways to further develop those strengths, and focus on the one significant challenge that often keeps them from being more effective. This process can have a profound impact on someone's development. This appreciative process encourages that the most time be spent on how to further develop natural strengths, which evidence shows is a more effective and sustaining approach than focusing on how to mitigate weaknesses (Buckingham & Clifton, 2001; Cooperrider, 2015; Gallup, 2013; Rath, 2007).

This appreciative process encourages that the most time be spent on how to further develop natural strengths, which evidence shows is a more effective and sustaining approach than focusing on how to mitigate weaknesses.

As discussed in the previous chapter, developing relational skills is approached differently from developing technical skills. Developing relational competence is supported by pausing and taking time for reflection. An example of how reflective practices can be built into busy health care settings is real-time coaching. A Michigan hospital wanted to help physicians improve their attuning behaviors—the most foundational of the relational practices—with patients. They created a process championed by a physician in their organization, in which coaches, identified from medicine, social work, and nursing, made rounds with physicians. After each patient encounter, the coach and physician paused just outside the room for about two minutes. They reflected on two simple questions: (1) What went well in the encounter? and (2) What would you have liked to have done differently? The purpose of the debriefing was to build relational awareness and attuning in real time. Some physicians initially felt uncomfortable with the prospect of having a coach shadow and debrief their patient visits, but the payoffs were so significant, including substantially improved patient satisfaction and improved sense of meaning in their work, that physicians began to seek out coaching.

Reviewing Individual Performance

When a goal of the organization is to advance relationship-based cultures, performance reviews need to reflect that goal. This can be achieved through the content of the performance reviews themselves. In a relationship-based culture, these reviews include opportunities to affirm the importance of relational competence by asking about it in ways that are informative and developmental while also holding employees accountable for their own relational competence. Human resources leaders, in partnership with executive leaders, can and must help set the strategic imperative for all performance reviews to advance the mission, vision, and values of the organization.

Helping Outliers Exit Gracefully

As we enhance our people selection and development processes, we will still encounter team members who don't fit the culture to which we aspire. Whether we're in an already established high-performing culture that is aspiring to be better or we're trying to establish a high-performing culture, we will face some people who don't (or won't) fit. This makes logical sense, yet we struggle with managing these folks off the team. Unfortunately, everyone else in the culture (including patients and families) suffers when we don't let these people go. In our experience, a pattern of inaction is a key barrier to improving or establishing a high-performing culture.

In a relationship-based culture, even the termination of a person's employment can be an opportunity for growth and development for everyone involved. Everything we say to and about the person must always be respectful, and the person's dignity must be safeguarded during the process. This respect comes more easily when we create a culture that believes that those released from employment are well-meaning and good human beings who simply have skill sets and attitudes that don't match the culture to which we aspire.

Building culture is ultimately every leader's job. Still, HR plays an essential role in accelerating this work and helping design the plan and systems to get there. The HR team is also central to making sure all of the organization's "people practices" are aligned with the broader goal of creating a high-performing enterprise. Progress toward this aim requires partnership, as do many things in health care: partnerships between the CEO and CHRO, HR leaders and hiring managers, physician leaders and administrative leaders, and there are many more examples. The first step on the journey to creating a high-performing organization is starting the conversation about what relational competence and a relationship-based culture can and must look like in your organization. Advancing a relationship-based culture requires HR leaders to create processes and systems that support and promote human connection and help individuals to optimize their potential.

Summary of Key Thoughts

- In relationship-based cultures, attuning, wondering, following, and holding must be embedded in every step of the talent life cycle—from recruitment to retirement or termination.

- Strong, healthy partnerships are essential to the success of every HR department and therefore of every organization.

- One of the primary benefits of the human resources business partner (HRBP) model is continuity of relationships, which allows HRBPs to become, over time, trusted advisors and objective coaches for the leaders they partner with, while also being their go-to resource for all things related to HR.

- It is essential to a relationship-based culture that all job postings be written in a way that demonstrates the level of relational competence we're looking for in team members. Additionally, all of our hiring processes must be relational as opposed to mechanical if we expect to attract people with a high aptitude for relational competence.

- New employees' onboarding experiences will set their expectations for culture going forward. What they experience in their onboarding process will make a bigger impression on them than anything that is said to them.

- Succession planning must include the identification of people who have the right technical skills for the roles an organization needs to fill. In a relationship-based culture, an additional focus is placed on identifying candidates who demonstrate high relational competence.

- In a relationship-based culture, performance reviews are central to building a developmental culture for all team members, and help people build their overall competency, including relational competence.

- Everyone in a health care culture, including patients and families, suffers when we make the choice to keep low performers or those who don't fit the culture in our organizations.

Reflection

- Reflect on the value of a healthy partnership between HR and operational leaders. Articulate the benefits of this close partnership for the organization and for individual employees.

- What are some ways that human resources professionals can support the development and assessment of relational competence in your organization?

- This chapter emphasizes the importance of having a highly relational process for those we recruit and hire. Discuss your process for communicating with people who have *not* been selected for hire. In what ways does your treatment of those people reflect a relationship-based culture? Why does it matter?

SECTION THREE
Teamwork and Interprofessional Practice

CHAPTER NINE
Relationship-Based Teaming

I think the extreme complexity of medicine has become more than an individual clinician can handle. But not more than teams of clinicians can handle.

ATUL GAWANDE

CHAPTER NINE

Relationship-Based Teaming

DONNA WRIGHT, ANN FLANAGAN PETRY, KARY GILLENWATERS,
AND DAVID ABELSON

In 1977, two Boeing jets collided on the Spanish island of Tenerife, killing 583 passengers. It was the deadliest accident in aviation history. Less than a year later, United Flight 173 crashed into suburban Portland, killing two crew members and eight passengers. The National Transportation Safety Board (NTSB) found that many factors contributed to these crashes, including a problem found in other crash investigations: Teams did not communicate well. Not only did the air traffic control team and cockpit crews misinterpret each other, but also, in the Portland crash, within the cockpit, the captain disregarded input from junior crewmembers, and junior crew members lacked the assertiveness to speak up.

Two years after these tragic crashes, the National Aeronautics and Space Administration (NASA) sponsored a conference highlighting its research of aviation accidents. The research pointed to the importance of human factors, including failures in communications, decision making, and leadership. In other words, suboptimal team functioning and cockpit culture contributed to significant loss of life (Helmreich, Merritt, & Wilhelm, 1999). Because of the NTSB investigations and NASA research, game-changing safety procedures and protocols were enacted.

Like aviation, health care is a life-and-death endeavor that has struggled with preventable errors. In 2000, the Institute of Medicine (IOM) released a landmark report: *To Err is Human: Building a Safer Health System*, which estimated that between 44,000 and 98,000 people die in hospitals each year due to preventable medical errors (Kohn et al., 2000). It offered a roadmap toward a safer health system.

Yet health care as an industry has been slower to embrace change than aviation has. Despite a huge increase in air travel over the past 20 years, the number of fatalities has fallen to all-time lows (Boeing, 2014). This stands in stark contrast to health care, in which analyses suggest that the IOM 1999 mortality figures underestimated preventable deaths. Studies published after 1999 estimate that 130,000–575,000 annual inpatient deaths are attributable to medical error. This is the equivalent of about three fatal airline crashes per day (Classen, 2011; Landrigan, 2010; Makary & Daniel, 2016; Sullenberger, 2013). What aviation and health care safety research reveals is that breakdowns in communication, not bad people or institutions (though institutional factors can contribute to bad communication), lead to lapses in safety.

Although patient harm from medical error does occur due to poor technical skill, lack of *relational,* not technical proficiency, is at the center of most medical errors and injuries (Kita, 2010; Makary, 2016; Moorthy, Munz, Adams, Pandey, & Darzi, 2005; Shanafelt, 2009; Yule, Flin, Paterson-Brown, Maran, & Rowley, 2006). It is sometimes hard to comprehend that relational skills override technical ability when it comes to overall team performance, but the evidence tells a powerful story.

Although patient harm from medical error does occur due to poor technical skill, lack of relational, not technical proficiency, is at the center of most medical errors and injuries.

Notably, studies by researchers at the Massachusetts Institute of Technology, Carnegie Mellon University, Harvard University, and elsewhere tell us what successful teams across all industries have in common. Most high-performing teams have two key ingredients. First, they have relational competencies, characterized by the ability to attune to others with empathy and sincerity (Goleman & Boyatzis, 2008; Koloroutis & Trout, 2012). Reliably successful teams can detect social cues, such as when someone is feeling upset or left out, and respond to them with curiosity and interest. On the other hand, people on ineffective teams are unable to do this with consistency and demonstrate far less sensitivity toward teammates (Woolley, Chabris, Pentland, Hashmi, & Malone, 2010). Second, in reliably successful teams, team members speak roughly the same amount—what social science researchers refer to as the equality in distribution of conversational turn-taking. Remarkably, if only one person or a small group speaks all the time, the collective intelligence of the team diminishes (Woolley, et al. 2010). These two important yet almost imperceptible practices create the conditions for psychological safety, respect, and open and honest communication (Duhigg, 2016; Edmundson, 2012; Goleman, 1998; Goleman & Boyatzis, 2008; Lieberman, 2013; Siegel, 2007). Indeed, these relational proficiencies are essential to achieving the best possible outcomes for patients and their loved ones.

In health care, relational competence is often an organizational blind spot. Yet it is every bit as important to continuously improve relational skills within teams as it is the structures and processes that undergird them. (See Appendix B for a list of relational core competencies tailored for teams.) The commitment to developing teams, then, takes a very special kind of relationship-based organization.

Teams Are Systems

Because teams are systems, they thrive or fail based on the quality of the interplay of the people, processes, and structures that comprise them. While we know that the processes and structures of teams are important (which is why there are countless books on those topics alone), we limit the scope of this chapter to the personal and interpersonal dimensions—the people component of teams. When teams are built around adequate processes and structures, it is the ability of team members to relate competently to the patient and family, as well as to one another, that becomes the make-or-break condition for quality, safety, and a good patient experience. This chapter focuses on the relational practices within the people component of teams.

It is the ability of team members to relate competently to the patient and family, as well as to one another, that is the make-or-break condition for quality, safety, and a good patient experience.

The People Component of Teams = "Teaming"

Good care happens when teams perform health care processes with reliability. People suffer unnecessarily and even die when teams don't perform these processes well. Healing occurs when teams—and not just the individuals on teams, but the teams themselves—hold patients and families in the center. This holding is complicated, of course, by the fact that teams continuously shape-shift based on need and circumstance. Further, the highly variable circumstances of illness create ambiguity about what is going on with a patient and uncertainty about the best course of action, which must be based partly on the values and preferences of patients.

How do we assure reliable care and compassionate holding in the face of necessarily complex processes and shape-shifting teams? And how do we foster adaptability in the face of the ambiguity, uncertainty, and rapidly changing circumstances of illness?

Amy Edmondson of the Harvard Business School, in her book *Teaming: How Organizations Learn, Innovate, and Compete in the Knowledge Economy*, defines teaming:

> Teaming is a verb. It is a dynamic activity, not a bounded, static entity. It is largely determined by the mindset and practices of teamwork, not by the design and structures of effective teams. Teaming is teamwork on the fly. It involves coordinating and collaborating without the benefit of stable team structures, because many operations, such as hospitals, power plants, and military installations, require a level of staffing flexibility that makes stable team composition rare. In a growing number of organizations, the constantly shifting nature of work means that many teams disband almost as soon as they've formed. You could be working on one team right now, but in a few days, or even a few minutes, you may be on another team. (Edmondson, 2012, p. 14)

In other words, the interpersonal aspect of teams requires defining *team* and *teaming* as verbs. We have seen that productive, efficient, compassionate teaming happens when attuning, wondering, following, and holding are used in interprofessional relationships.

Applying Attuning, Wondering, Following, and Holding for Effective Teaming

When we use attuning, wondering, following, and holding with patients and families, we refer to them as *therapeutic practices*. When we use them with our team members (and our friends and loved ones, for that matter), we call them *relational practices*. The remainder of this chapter will explore how the application of the four relational practices improves relationships among team members and therefore team functioning. We will examine the application of each practice in turn.

Attuning

> Attuning is the practice of being present in the moment and "tuning in" to team members.

Attunement arises from our brain's natural capacity to relate with others. When we attune with compassion, we are harnessing our innate human inclination for meaningful connection. Nearly all people share this remarkable capacity and yearn for human connection. Attunement is vital because it creates a felt sense of connection. Without it, team members feel disjointed and communication is less coherent; under these conditions, meaning and purpose are often lost. Remarkably, many teams function in a disjointed, disorganized way simply because they are unaware of just how pivotal attunement is to team communication and team efficacy. Compassionate attuning is the interpersonal process that enables people to have meaningful interactions and to feel moved to act on another's behalf. It is, therefore, essential to healthy teams.

Reflection on Interprofessional Teaming with Stellar Results

> Imagine working at Children's National Health System in Washington, D.C., where staff members regularly care for kids who are in crisis. In fact, the term *children with medical complexity* (CMC) is all too familiar. That term was used to describe Leah (not her real name), an eight-year-old Children's National patient. She has severe autism; some of her symptoms include becoming highly distressed by

unfamiliar people and stimuli, and she has difficulty communicating. Having accompanied her to numerous therapies and doctor visits, her parents are deeply knowledgeable about her care. They just don't happen to have a formal clinical title, as the other members of her care team do. For example, there is a neurologist, gastroenterologist, and an anesthesiologist, but the team at Children's National understand that Leah's parents are Leah-*ologists*. So, when Leah was diagnosed with Crohn's disease, the interprofessional team ensured that there were representatives on the team who touched all aspects of Leah's care, including her parents.

Fortunately, Leah and her family had the benefit of a highly technically skilled team who compassionately tuned in to her unique needs while also tuning in to how different members of the team might be able to meet those needs. The whole team—Leah's parents included—considered the best way to provide a regimen of infusions, usually given in an outpatient clinic. Even though this was a terrifying option because of Leah's reactivity to the unfamiliar, the team compassionately moved forward with treatment. They customized care as best they could, but despite their efforts, treatment proved traumatic. Because of the cohesive, highly attuned relationship the team created with one another, Leah's parents spoke up right away, and there was honest dialogue about other options.

Undeterred and on a mission to help Leah, the team tried inpatient infusions. Even with a more specialized approach, this too was traumatic and overwhelming. The team paused to attune to one another again and ultimately came up with a novel plan: infusions, along with non-operating room anesthesia (NORA). Along the way, the care team invited people from multiple specialty groups onto the team to provide care unrelated to Crohn's but that would also require sedation, such as dental and skin care. Leah's mother performed routine personal hygiene including facial, nail, and ear care while Leah was under anesthesia, and her father was permitted to gownup and hold her hand as she was going under and coming out of anesthesia. In another accommodation, the nurse navigator and anesthesiologist met the family in a parking garage and partnered with the security department to clear halls and elevators to travel to the NORA room, thus limiting environmental stressors and triggers. The collaboration led to the most innovative clinical interventions and significantly reduced avoidable suffering and post-traumatic memories for Leah, her parents, and the staff.

The real power of teamwork lies in the way people come together and tune in to one another to fulfill a shared purpose. Teams everywhere, including those at Children's National, have the potential to be catalysts of hope and healing for patients in crisis. To be sure, in Leah's care, there were vital structures and processes in place that created the conditions for the best

> *Teams have the potential to be catalysts of hope and healing for patients in crisis.*

outcomes to emerge. Within that fortunate context, people spoke up, took all perspectives into account, and weren't afraid to try new approaches. The team's ability to attune to one another, listen to what mattered most to the family, and adjust with each new episode of care revealed the team's relational competence, as well as their commitment to the best possible technical care. As you can imagine, this sort of highly attuned teaming has a tremendously positive effect on the culture. This event even led to the creation of a new nurse navigator role in the organization, allowing this example of seamless teamwork to become the norm.

Wondering

Wondering is the practice of being genuinely interested in team members, including what each person can contribute. It requires an openhearted curiosity about what can be learned from each individual, while intentionally suspending assumptions and judgment.

The term *wondering* might seem distinctly nonclinical, but when we bring a mindset of wondering to teamwork, especially in patient care, it is a profoundly effective clinical tool. Take, for example, the experience of a team member raising a concern about a patient in a busy clinic or emergency department. We may initially be annoyed, thinking, "I don't have time for this," but the decision to wonder, as opposed to quickly judging the suggestion to be insignificant, can mean the difference between life and death.

As team members, wondering can also mean pausing to consider whether we have all the needed voices on the team.

Reflection on Occupational Therapy as a Member of the Team

Louise was 75 years old and had multiple medical conditions; her health history included two heart attacks and breast cancer, and she was currently dealing with leukemia, dizzy spells, heart failure, macular degeneration, and anxiety. She was hospitalized 58 times in one year with complaints seemingly related to any and all of these conditions; no known etiology was found for her symptoms.

When Dora, a home health aide, visited Louise to assist her with bathing after a recent hospitalization, she was surprised to find her at the sink doing dishes with her adult granddaughter, Natalie. Louise's husband, seated with a cup of coffee, said to her, "Louise, why don't you sit down and let Natalie wash the dishes." Louise replied tearfully, "What do you want me to do—nothing?" He was perplexed, and Dora was deeply aware that Louise's exasperation was not about the dishes.

After helping Louise with her bath (which Louise clearly did not want help with), Dora found a moment to ask Natalie how her grandmother was doing. Natalie told her that along with all of her medical diagnoses, Louise was experiencing social isolation due to a weakened immune system and that this was a big loss for her. She used to go for coffee with friends, work outside the home, and travel regularly to visit family who lived several states away. Her isolation also compromised her spiritual life, as she could no longer attend daily Mass. She had long prided herself on her ability to make a house a home, waking at 4:45 a.m. and not going to bed until 11 p.m. in order to do all the things that kept up a home, but now a person was coming in several times a week to clean, do the laundry—to do *her* work. Without the ability to be of service to the people she loved, she felt that her life lacked purpose, and her health and wellbeing were impacted by her diminished sense of worth. Dora could see clearly why none of Louise's hospitalizations could fix that, and she had an idea about who might be able to help.

Dora called Louise's clinic and got Natalie a phone consultation with an occupational therapist (OT). Natalie and the OT discussed Louise's situation in detail and came up with the following plan: (1) the person who helped with housekeeping would include Louise in whatever way her energy level could allow, (2) a nun would visit her weekly and bring communion and also call her for a brief phone visit at the same time every day (she thrived on routine), and (3) another volunteer visitor happened to have a counseling background, so he could easily recognize her tendency to get stuck in her thoughts of anxiety and help steer their conversations onto more enjoyable subjects.

The result of this plan was zero hospitalizations in the following three years. Before this intervention, during each of Louise's 58 hospital admissions, each member of the team had done an excellent job of assessing everything they were supposed to assess and treating everything they were supposed to treat. Their goal was to get her back to what they knew as her baseline and to get her home. The problem was not that any members of the team failed to do their jobs; the problem was that before there was an OT on the team, it was no one's job to focus entirely on how Louise's daily activities could improve her overall health. The sort of creative problem solving the OT used to help restore Louise's quality of life is a skill that is not exclusive to OTs. It is, however, every OT's specialty; that's what OTs do. Occupational therapists ask questions nobody else is likely to ask, and they are masters at coming up with small solutions that solve big problems.

Willingness to pause and wonder about whether we have the right players on the team is fundamental to team effectiveness. Particularly in instances in which problems, challenges, and crises persist (as they did in Leah's and Louise's cases), it's important for teams to take time to wonder together about who can be added to the team in order to save them time and save their patients unnecessary suffering, in the long run. Any time we're faced with frequent readmissions or "nonadherence" to treatment, that's a cue to get curious and wonder about who we might be missing on the team.

Following

Following is the practice of listening to and focusing on what a team member is teaching us about what matters most to her and allowing that information to guide our interactions with her.

When you recall the feeling of being part of an amazing team, do you recall members who were particularly gifted at creating an environment for the team to do their best work? Perhaps they emerged as ad hoc leaders. They may have cultivated an energizing team culture in subtle ways, perhaps by demonstrating genuine interest in each person. They listened to what each person had to say; they were curious about each team member's thoughts and feelings; and they noticed if someone was quiet or being talked over, and steered team dialogue toward more balanced participation. They may have been a sounding board, helping the team reflect on processes or interactions. They may have demonstrated what it looks like to offer a trustworthy ear, even when team members expressed raw, awkward emotions such as fear, shame, or grief. These are examples of what "following" behaviors can look like in team settings.

We are all more likely to thrive with the support of someone who listens and brings out the best in a team, perhaps seeing potential the team didn't see in itself. Team members follow when they take an active interest in one another's opinions. Diverse opinions emerge when people feel it is safe to speak up and that others care about their perspective. Relationally adept teams explicitly embrace diverse opinions, encouraging conversational turn-taking, as well as allowing for the silence of those who participate best by listening intently without comment. Team norms reinforce the value of following each member and following the team as a whole. Following was demonstrated by Leah's care team when they listened to her parents' input, embracing them as members of the care team, and adapted treatment plans to reduce suffering for Leah. Following enabled the team to more quickly learn from one another and to learn as a team.

Holding

Holding is the practice of intentionally creating psychological safety within the team by demonstrating respect and caring and by supporting conversational turn-taking.

Holding can be described as verbal and nonverbal behaviors that communicate unconditional warm regard and nonjudgment toward another.

When we talk about team trust and psychological safety, two main types of trust are in play. The first is role-based trust, which means we assume that the individual within a process has the training, scope of practice, judgment, and skills to perform competently. It means, "I trust that you know your job and that you will do it to the best of your ability." Role-based trust assumes that people within their roles will act to the limit of their scope of practice and fulfill their responsibilities.

The second is interpersonal trust, which can be defined as having mutual respect and concern for one another. Meaningful interpersonal interactions require interpersonal trust. This kind of trust can be expressed as, "I trust that I can count on you as a person." Psychological safety—the sense that one will not be belittled, attacked, or ignored—is the bedrock of interpersonal trust. When interpersonal trust is high, people feel that it is safe to express vulnerability through such actions as asking for and accepting help or raising concerns on behalf of the patient and family.

Notably, interpersonal trust has a stronger positive correlation with team performance than role-based trust (Webber, 2008). Therefore, integrating

Within a holding environment, team members learn, discover insights, and gracefully recover from mistakes.

behaviors that communicate nonjudgmental holding are critical to health care team performance.

Within a holding environment, team members learn, discover insights, and gracefully recover from mistakes. When errors happen or omissions are made, it can take a terrible toll on everyone. The increase in burnout, addiction, and suicide point to the impact on providers as the "second victims" of medical mistakes (Wu, 2000). There is no question that the patient and family are the primary focus, but when health care professionals make mistakes, they are often traumatized and suffer silently. The key is for teams to offer a safe space for one another in which to talk about and learn from mistakes. Learning is lost if people feel they will be punished and judged harshly.

A team mindset of unconditional warm regard does not mean that everyone on the team likes everyone else or enjoys their company. It means they hold each person with respect, kindness, and the acknowledgment that they are human too. They suffer too. They have insecurities, wounds, and fears just like we do, and they want to feel valued and appreciated just like we do.

Additionally, holding another with unconditional regard doesn't mean we condone recklessness or enable failure to learn. On the contrary, it means we explicitly socialize teaming behaviors that foster accountability, caring, direct language, displaying vulnerability, inviting participation, and acknowledging our limits.

This chapter began with a reflection on how people in the field of aviation learned the importance of psychological safety as a condition for team members to speak up. Role-based trust, combined with interpersonal trust as a team norm, creates psychological safety. Prior to "crew resource management," a set of training procedures for use in environments in which human error can have devastating effects, cockpit culture resembled health care, with pilots and physicians at the tops of their respective hierarchies. Lacking interpersonal trust, cockpit crew members feared speaking up and disagreeing with the pilot. Similarly, if interpersonal trust is lacking in a health care team, members hesitate to question physicians and others. Indeed, over the years, we have observed teams so devoid of interpersonal trust that one physician would not question another.

Analyses of cockpit voice recordings from crashes prior to crew resource management revealed instances of cockpit crewmembers indirectly attempting to give pilots critical but conflicting information. These veiled attempts failed because of the cockpit culture, which was low in interpersonal trust, and fatal crashes ensued.

This risky behavior of indirect communication occurs in health care as well. Medical residents may be working side by side with nurses or other team members who have more years of clinical experience. These team members sometimes "tiptoe," employing indirect, veiled language because of perceived role hierarchy. Tiptoeing is a sure sign of insufficient interpersonal trust. A more effective environment for any new clinician is one in which mentoring and coaching across disciplines is the norm. This kind of culture allows new team members to drop the façade of perfection and invulnerability in exchange for psychological safety and shared learning within the team.

Health care organizations do best when, as in aviation, they embrace both the technical and the human dimensions of improving processes.

This all has an effect on patients and families as well. In health care, when both role-based trust and interpersonal trust are high, the team fulfills a third trust— the trust that patients and families place in the team. The trust they have in us is rarely *Disengaged team members destroy holding because you can catch only so much with a broken net.* articulated, and it may not be based on anything beyond the logistics of the current situation. Consider this analogy: If you were falling from a high cliff, and the group of people below included firefighters, you'd trust the firefighters to figure out how to catch you or at least to give you the softest landing possible. In health care, people are sometimes just that vulnerable; when they're not literally falling into our arms, they're still trusting us to catch them, no matter what happens, or at least to break their fall. This is why healthy teaming is so important. If one member of a team is just showing up and doing tasks but isn't really part of the team, that person is putting a *hole* in the team, through which the patient and family may eventually fall. Disengaged team members destroy holding because you can catch only so much with a broken net.

The noble cause of health care provides all of us with a responsibility to honor the trust extended to us by patients, their families, and the communities we serve. It is a hope-filled trust. They trust us to hold their wellbeing in the center of all we do. Our job—our privilege—is to do everything in our power to fulfill the inherent trust extended to us by every person who comes into our care.

Summary of Key Thoughts

- Quality and safety in health care depend on healthy team relationships.

- When communication—both interprofessional and within a single discipline—feels unsafe to anyone on the team, patients, families, teams, and organizations suffer preventable harm.

- Lack of relational proficiency is at the center of most medical errors and injuries.

- Through studying the equality in distribution of conversational turn taking, social scientists have determined that all team members on high-functioning teams speak roughly the same amount.

- Relational competence is often an organizational blind spot, yet it is every bit as important to continuously improve relational skills within teams as it is the structures and processes which undergird them.

- Healing occurs when teams hold patients and families in the center of their care.

- "Teaming is teamwork on the fly. It involves coordinating and collaborating without the benefit of stable team structures, because many operations, such as hospitals, power plants, and military installations, require a level of staffing flexibility that makes stable team composition rare" (Edmondson, 2012, p. 14).

- Attuning is the practice of being present in the moment and "tuning in" to team members. Compassionate attuning is the interpersonal process that enables people to have meaningful interactions and to feel moved to act on another's behalf. Attunement is essential to healthy teams.

- Wondering is the practice of being genuinely interested in our fellow team members. As team members, wondering can also mean pausing to consider whether we have all the necessary people on the team.

- Following is the practice of listening to and focusing on what team members are teaching us about what matters most to them. We are all more likely to thrive with the support of someone who listens and brings out the best in the team— perhaps seeing potential in the team that the team didn't see in itself.

- Holding is the practice of intentionally creating psychological safety within the team by demonstrating respect and caring and supporting conversational turn taking.

- Role-based trust means we assume that the individual within a process has the training, scope of practice, judgment, and skills to perform competently. Role-based trust means, "I trust that you know your job and that you will do it to the best of your ability."

- Interpersonal trust can be defined as having mutual respect and concern for one another. Meaningful interpersonal interactions require interpersonal trust.

- The noble cause of health care provides all of us with a responsibility to honor the trust extended to us by patients, their families, and the communities we serve. It is a hope-filled trust.

Reflection

- Quality and safety in care depend on healthy team relationships. Describe a time when your team learned from a mistake and identified improvements, including improvements in team relationships and communication.

- What strikes you about "teaming"—the idea that teams often form "on the fly" rather than existing as stable teams—as a particular challenge in health care? What systems or processes have helped you build a sense of cohesion and trust in your ever-changing teams?

- Psychological safety is fundamental to healthy teamwork. Discuss times in which members of the team spoke up on behalf of the patient, even when it was uncomfortable. In what ways was that supported or not?

- Given that occupational therapists are so skilled at finding small solutions for large problems, could it be that occupational therapists are health care's secret resource for cost containment? What are some ways that OTs could automatically become members of teams in your organization?

- This chapter ends with the idea that the "noble cause" of health care provides all of us with a responsibility to honor the trust extended to us by patients, their families, and the communities we serve. Describe ways in which this responsibility informs your team's work and relationships on a daily basis.

SECTION FOUR
Patient Care Delivery and Systems Thinking

CHAPTER TEN
Care Delivery Design that Holds Patients and Families

Every system is perfectly designed to get the results it gets.

W. EDWARDS DEMING

CHAPTER TEN

Care Delivery Design that Holds Patients and Families

SUSAN WESSEL, DAVID ABELSON, AND MARIE MANTHEY

Steve Jobs, the cofounder of Apple and former CEO of Pixar, died in 2011 from a rare form of pancreatic cancer. During the course of his relatively short life, Jobs transformed multiple industries, including personal computing with the Apple II, animated movies with Pixar, the music industry with the iPod and iTunes, mobile phones with the iPhone, and publishing and tablet computers with the iPad. In 2010, *Forbes* estimated his net worth at $6 billion and ranked him as the 17th most powerful person in the world, several positions ahead of Nicolas Sarkozy, then president of France.

After his grave diagnosis, he benefited from receiving cutting-edge health care technology, including a liver transplant. He was one of the first people in the world to have all of the genes of his cancer tumor, as well as of his normal DNA, sequenced. It was a process that cost more than $100,000.

But his billions could not buy care coordination.

Jobs' authorized biographer describes how the wife of the 17th most powerful person in the world needed to assume responsibility for coordinating his care:

> Jobs allowed his wife to convene a meeting of his doctors. He realized he was facing the type of problem that he never permitted at Apple. His treatment was fragmented rather than integrated.

Each of his myriad maladies was being treated by different special-ists—oncologists, pain specialists, nutritionists, hepatologists and hematologists—but they were not being coordinated in a cohesive approach ... "One of the big issues in the health care industry is the lack of caseworkers or advocates that are the quarterback of each team," Powell [Jobs' wife] said. This was particularly true at Stanford, where nobody seemed in charge of figuring out how nutrition was related to pain care and to oncology. So Powell asked the various Stanford specialists to come to their house for a meeting ... They agreed on a new program regimen for dealing with the pain and coor-dinating the other treatments. (Isaacson, 2015, pp. 549–550)

Jobs, with all of his wealth, could not purchase coordinated care because his care was not designed to be coordinated. One can imagine that an invitation from the seventeenth most powerful person in the world is not to be ignored. Unfortunately, patients and families with less power (i.e., the rest of us) must rely on organizations to design care that is safe and effective and that holds us compassionately in the center.

The Importance of Effective Care Delivery Design

Good care delivery design results in the safest possible care with the best possible outcomes while patients and families experience being held. Poor design has the potential to result in unintended outcomes, avoidable human suffering, and unnecessary deaths.

The word *deliver* (*Merriam-Webster's*: to take something to a person or place) suggests a one-way transaction between sender and receiver rather than a two-way interaction between partners. Senders send; recipients receive. We prefer an alternative definition of *deliver*: to do what you say you will do or what people expect you to do; to produce the promised, wanted, or expected result.

Good care delivery design results in the safest possible care with the best possible outcomes while patients and families experience being held.

Thus, delivery of care is about organizations continuously improving their systems to deliver on their promise to provide the best possible care outcomes. The Institute of Medicine (IOM, 2001) proposes a summary of the domains of expectations for delivery: care that is safe, effective, patient centered, timely, efficient, and equitable. Rather than inventory the many studies showing the gaps in U.S. health care in these domains and the many useful approaches to narrowing these gaps, this chapter focuses on three simple rules of care delivery design that we believe can be distilled from the studies. These simple rules—hold the patient and family, make the best way the easiest way, and support all relationships—establish guidelines for creating the optimal system to deliver care in every setting.

An everyday example illustrates the complexity facing care delivery design. Consider the experience of an elderly man who needs a bladder procedure that will require an inpatient stay after surgery. In addition to his primary care physician, he sees a cardiologist for heart failure, a nephrologist for poor kidney function, an endocrinologist for diabetes, a pulmonary physician for chronic obstructive pulmonary disease, a physical therapist for back pain, and a nurse care manager for diabetes and heart failure. In other words, prior to hospitalization, this man is involved in multiple care episodes involving dozens of teams and hundreds of people. Additionally, during his hospitalization, he will have many more interactions with clinicians in multiple roles involving complex and potentially dangerous processes such as anesthesia.

How does a care delivery system assure that this elderly man (who is also a husband, parent, grandparent, and artist) feels safely held during his bladder surgery that will span weeks from the initial evaluation to the last postoperative checkup? And how can the system most reliably deliver the best possible clinical outcomes for the surgery? How does a care delivery system hold this elderly man and his family as weeks pass following the surgery? Who will this patient and family turn to if they experience complications? How do they *know* whom to turn to? Who accepts responsibility for holding this man's whole experience? Good care delivery design means there are ready responses to all of these questions, using simple rules to improve complex systems.

Good care delivery design also means that the designers of care create systems in which every subsystem, process, and structure allows all of the people involved to connect with each other as people. Good care delivery design means that there is an organization-wide commitment to attune to the experience of care through the eyes of the patient and family.

Three Simple Rules for Highly Attuned Care Delivery Systems

Complex adaptive systems, such as care delivery, can be viewed as emerging from a handful of simple rules applied over and over. Thus, students of complex systems recommend working to improve the attributes of a system by defining a few simple rules that can be embedded everywhere (Plsek, 2001).

We propose the following three simple rules to advance relationship-based care delivery design:

1. Hold the patient and family.

2. Make the best way the easiest way.

3. Support all relationships.

We believe that designing the delivery system using these simple rules actively promotes the conditions for care that is safe, effective, patient centered, timely, efficient, and equitable. What follows is a closer look at how each rule can be actualized as part of a care delivery system.

Rule 1: Hold the Patient and Family

Care delivery design begins with the patient and family in mind. The British National Health Service articulates this as, "No decision about me without me." This means that all design is approached through the lens of what it will mean for the patient and family, including ease of access, prevention of complications, smooth transitions, and reduction of suffering. We cannot presume to know what is best without being attuned to the patient's and family's perspective. This means seeking their perspective and involving them along the entire design process, including evaluating the current system, prioritizing improvements, designing changes, identifying and evaluating measures of success, and planning further refinements. As was evident in the story in the Teaming chapter about Leah, the eight-year-old girl with severe autism for whom many processes were customized, the team's ability to embrace the family as a source of information is essential to the team's success. Patients and families become our expert go-to source for how our systems are working.

Patients and families become our expert go-to source for how our systems are working.

Application of Rule 1: Use Language that Holds Patients and Families

Holding the patient and family includes sensitivity to how language reflects and shapes attitudes. Our language can reinforce the personhood of the individual, or it can cause us to see the person as an object (workload, a diagnosis, a label, or an obstacle). Therefore, it is important to cultivate a culture in which we are mindful of our language. Speaking about people in a way that preserves their dignity, whether they are present or not, is a way of holding.

The language we use can and will change our behavior and the behavior of others. Consider the difference between "This patient is in pain and her daughter is very demanding—you'd better be prepared!" and "This daughter is very anxious about her mom's condition, and she is the primary caregiver at home. She needs support and reassurance—perhaps some ideas about resources." Our language can set people up for successful connection, or it can encourage bias and a failure to wonder. This organizational value of holding patients and families must be clear and explicit, and it comes right from the heart of every patient: "Say nothing about me that you wouldn't say in front of me." Here are some questions teams can explore together to facilitate awareness of language:

- Do our words consistently convey dignity and respect for the personhood of each patient and family?

- Does the way we convey information about the patient in our notes and in our team communication demonstrate attuning and wondering?

- Do we have areas of bias or blind spots that are revealed through our language?

- What are some ways our language may objectify the patient or family?

- What are ways we respect and hold our patients in our use of language?

Application of Rule 1: Design Transitions that Hold the Patient

Transitions between care settings, such as referral from the primary care clinician to specialists or discharge from the hospital, represent a critical time when patients may experience "falling through the cracks" rather than feeling held. Applying a mindset that makes *holding the patient and family* an explicit goal during transitions means the system is designed so that the professional team is considering subsequent interactions and preparing the patient, family, and future teams. This is as important in ambulatory settings as it is in inpatient settings.

Systems and processes should be designed such that when a subsequent team is ready for a patient, the patient immediately feels known. Coincidentally, preparing patients, families, and care teams for subsequent interactions also exemplifies Rule 2, *make the best way the easiest way.* Being prepared is the best way; being prepared is easier than not being prepared.

Far too often, health care professionals don't fully appreciate that the vast majority of chronic disease care does not occur within the walls of the health care organization, but instead takes place at home, work, and school, and is carried out by the patient, sometimes assisted by family and friends. This reality points to the importance of designing care in partnership with those who will assume the care outside the walls of the clinic or hospital. Often, poor communication or lack of understanding of the challenges faced by families and clinicians providing care outside the clinic or hospital results in disruption in the coordination, efficiency, and effectiveness of care. This can be especially true during times of transition and are of particular concern for patients coping with chronic illness. Holding through transition to home includes preparation pertaining to medications, diet, activity, criteria for returning to the formal health care delivery system, and assessment for the status of chronic diseases such as diabetes, hypertension, and heart failure.

Rule 2: Make the Best Way the Easiest Way

The staggering complexity of modern health care exceeds the capacity of the unaided human mind to navigate, let alone master it. Nearly 70,000 discrete diagnoses exist, along with more than 70,000 named medical procedures (CDC, 2015). In 2014, the International Association of Scientific, Technical, and Medical Publishers (STM) reported that researchers published 2.5 million articles in 34,550 peer-reviewed journals (Ware & McCabe, 2015). Now add the complexity of insurance coverage minutia and the many different providers, locations, and agencies that might be involved in any one case. It is within this context that patients may have to interact with complex processes associated with scheduling, registration, admission, discharge, order entry, imaging, lab, medications, blood products, anesthesia, billing, benefit assessment, insurance coverage, homecare needs, challenges with activities of daily living, surgery, and physical therapy, to name just a few. Making the best way the easiest way gives us a grounding principle to help mitigate this dizzying complexity.

Application of Rule 2: Maximize the Invaluable Resource of the People Closest to the Work

The efficiency and effectiveness of care delivery design are maximized when the people closest to the work are involved in creating and revising their own systems. The reasons are simple: No one knows the work better, and if people are engaged in innovating the design, they will feel more ownership for the work, making them more eager to participate in subsequent improvements. We know from countless implementations of Relationship-Based Care (RBC) that the engagement of first-line staff is critical to the creation of efficient systems within care delivery design. *The Relationship-Based Care Field Guide* explains how unit practice councils

(UPCs) gather first-line staff members into the work of amending their processes and structures to keep patients and families in the center of their care (Koloroutis et al., 2007, pp. 214–216). The tacit goal of every UPC is always to make the best way the easiest way.

Application of Rule 2: Make It Crystal Clear Who's Responsible for What

An essential aspect of making the best way the easiest way is ensuring that all team members are:

- clear about their roles

- provided with enough clarity to take ownership for their full scope of responsibility, authority, and accountability

- supported in practicing to their full capacity

Interventions such as Creative Health Care Management's Role Clarity and Work Alignment process can be used to (1) determine the character of work activities of all providers for a specific population of patients, and (2) identify the complexity of the interventions routinely performed. Interventions of this sort provide a clear, comprehensive picture of how each department functions so that changes in roles, policies, processes, and procedures can be based on relevant, timely data about what there is to do and who there is to do it.

Along with role clarity, it is very helpful for teams to have a common language to use when discussing who is responsible for what actions, who has decision-making authority and for which patients, and who is ultimately accountable in any given situation.

Responsibility + Authority + Accountability, often shortened to R+A+A, is a practical formula to facilitate greater personal ownership and alignment with and among teams (Creative Health Care Management, 2003; Koloroutis, 2004; Manthey, 2002, 2007). When teams are not functioning in the ways they are intended to function, it is likely that one or more of these three components is out of balance. Most typically, someone is asked to take responsibility and full accountability but is not given the authority necessary to achieve what she's taken responsibility for.

Here is the R+A+A formula spelled out:

- **Responsibility:** The clear allocation and acceptance of one's duties and obligations so that everyone knows who is responsible for what and when.

- **Authority:** The right to act in the area for which one has been allocated and has accepted responsibility. Four levels of authority apply to patient care:

  Level 1: Authority to inform

  Level 2: Authority to recommend

  Level 3: Authority to communicate, collaborate, and then act

  Level 4: Authority to act independently

  The appropriate level of authority is based on the scope of responsibility of a person or group. Clarification of which level applies is functionally useful.

- **Accountability:** The retrospective review of the decisions made or actions taken to determine if they were appropriate, so that, if they were not appropriate, corrective action can be taken, which must be developmental rather than punitive.

In all of our RBC implementations, using the language of R+A+A helps people get right to the core of the majority of problems encountered in care delivery.

Application of Rule 2: Design Processes and Structures that Minimize Reliance on Human Memory

Because of the complexity of illness in health care, Rule 2 compels us to design systems that minimize reliance on human memory in order to free up the cognition of clinicians for judgment and critical thinking. When our design includes easy-to-navigate structures and processes and excellent care coordination, it is both easiest and best for everyone involved. The efficiencies that result also free up more time to build relationships with colleagues, patients, and families. This design rule doesn't apply only to our own care processes. It applies to the processes and structures we create for patients and families to navigate.

Good care delivery design embeds the "usual best approach" as the default mode, often using the electronic health record (EHR) for evidence-based order sets, documentation templates, and reminders for things such as medication interactions and adverse reactions, or preventive services that are due. The aim is to make the best way a path of least resistance. Clinicians may override the default mode, but it takes a bit more work. Designing cylinders of anesthesia so that it's impossible to affix a tube to the wrong valve is a classic example of error proofing independent of checklists, and it's an ideal example of making the best way the easiest way.

When our design includes easy-to-navigate structures and processes and excellent care coordination, it is both easiest and best for everyone involved.

Application of Rule 2: Make Care Coordination a Priority

Care coordination involves embedding the best way as the easiest way in both our structures and our processes. As an example, care delivery organizations generally adopt the academic model of grouping similar specialties together rather than organizing care around problems that involve multiple specialties. As a result, patients and families sometimes feel like pinballs careening from one specialty to another in order to obtain a coherent diagnosis and treatment plan for problems like gait imbalance, prostate cancer, or musculoskeletal symptoms that span multiple specialties. Contrast this with an alternative structure that groups specialties, diagnostic tests, and therapeutic procedures for discrete problems into centers or "institutes." Examples include musculoskeletal centers with orthopedic surgeons, imaging, physical therapy, pharmacies, and operating suites, or dedicated centers for thyroid surgery bringing together endocrinologists, head and neck surgeons, and thyroid imaging. In this way, all the varied expertise needed for the care of these patients is available in one location rather than the patient having to travel to numerous locations.

Making the best way the easiest way for care coordination also involves matching the appropriate coordination strategies with the level of need. Care coordination needs can be visualized as a pyramid, with each layer building upon and adding to the previous layer as the patient's needs become more complex. (See Figure 10.1.)

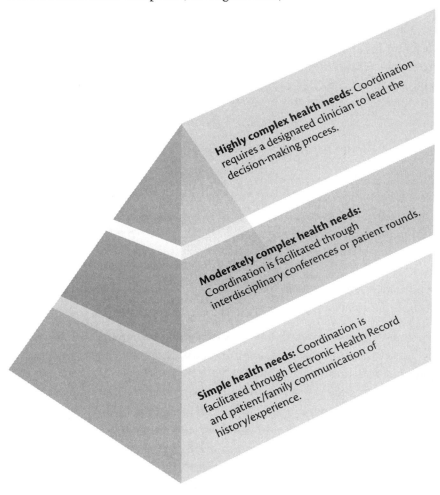

Highly complex health needs: Coordination requires a designated clinician to lead the decision-making process.

Moderately complex health needs: Coordination is facilitated through interdisciplinary conferences or patient rounds.

Simple health needs: Coordination is facilitated through Electronic Health Record and patient/family communication of history/experience.

Figure 10.1: Pyramid of Care Coordination Strategies

The base of this pyramid represents most of the population—those who are largely healthy and have episodic needs met in their primary care settings. For this group, coordination is usually facilitated through an integrated EHR along with the patient or family providing a cogent history. In moderately complex patient situations, represented in the middle tier of the pyramid, coordination is best facilitated through interdisciplinary collaboration during care conferences or rounds. At the apex of the pyramid, when complexity and uncertainty abound and professionals may disagree, a designated clinician is empowered to lead a collaborative decision-making process and reach decisions with the patient and family. Effective collaboration involves intentional relationships and a common mission. Each member must be willing to share autonomy while maintaining their separate identities as professionals (Winer & Ray, 1994).

Rule 3: Support All Relationships

Effective care delivery systems operationalize the four relational practices (attuning, wondering, following, and holding) within the three key relationships (self, colleagues, patients/families). Applying Rule 3 to care delivery design means designing processes and structures that promote continuity of clinician-patient relationships and interprofessional collaboration.

Application of Rule 3: Cultivate Ownership and Continuity of Relationships through a System of Primary Clinicians

Rule 3—support all relationships—necessitates that care delivery be designed to maximize the continuity of clinicians' relationships with patients and families so that the patient and family feel an increased sense of safety and being known. This design also encourages each clinician's sense of ownership for each patient relationship.

Primary Nursing is a care delivery system that emphasizes continuity of care and acceptance of responsibility of care by a named RN over a period of time (Manthey, 2002; Person, 2004; Wessel & Manthey, 2015). The Primary Nursing system has been preferred in hospital settings and is also of high value in primary care and specialty clinics, homecare settings, telemedicine, hospice, and long-term care. The principles of Primary Nursing have also been applied by clinicians in other professional disciplines and in support services (Wessel & Manthey, 2015). The key tenet of a delivery system with primary relationships is that while the

The Primary Nursing system has been preferred in hospital settings and is also of high value in primary care and specialty clinics, homecare settings, telemedicine, hospice, and long-term care.

system design expects and supports *all* team members to know and hold patients and families, a named primary clinician within each discipline accepts responsibility for knowing the patient and family as people, for learning and sharing what's important to them, for planning the care provided by their discipline, and for collaborating with the rest of the team to integrate and coordinate care.

While it's not surprising that continuity of relationships and the resulting increased sense of ownership result in a culture in which patients and families feel held and all relationships are supported, it also makes the best way the easiest way. In *Primary Nursing: Person-Centered Care Delivery System Design,* Heidi Nolen, BSN, RN, a primary nurse at UC Davis Medical Center, explains why:

> There may be a time when I have four primary patients on the unit, and I wonder whether I'll be capable of caring for all of them because of the acuity. A lot of times, for me personally, even with the acuity, I'd be more open to taking care of those patients I've had as primaries before because I already know them and that's half the battle. Sometimes half the challenge of being busy is just not knowing the family dynamics or their preferences, so I would still rather care for them even if the acuity was higher because I've already established the relationship ... As soon as the family trusts you, the whole dynamic changes. They feel a calmness with you, and you feel it with them, and you can just go directly to your job without having to explain as many things because you've already established the trust factor and the relationship is formed. If you can build the trust and the relationship, it just makes even the hardest days easier. (Wessel & Manthey, 2015, pp. 6, 114)

Continuity of relationships is particularly important when caring for people with complex, chronic conditions. Proactive communication and easy access to a person who can take timely action when needed can prevent both complications and unnecessary hospitalization. Primary relationships facilitate such proactivity and responsiveness. The key to building a high level of patient and family trust in inpatient settings and for people living with chronic conditions is to provide clarity about which *one person* is responsible for building the relationship and making decisions with them about their plan for care. The person responsible for the primary relationship then coordinates and integrates their plan with the plans of other members of the interprofessional team. Such a system of primary clinicians has proven effective in improving clinician-patient relationships and facilitating care decisions that achieve the patient's goals.

Primary care settings have been known for continuity of the physician-patient relationship over time and for valuing the role of patient as partner. An example of this is the Patient-Centered Medical Home model (Peikes, Genevro, Scholle, & Torda, 2011), which prioritizes primary relationships in ambulatory care. These authors describe a patient-centered medical home as a way of organizing primary care that emphasizes care coordination and communication to transform primary care into "what patients want it to be" (NCQA, 2016). Each patient has an ongoing relationship with a physician, a nurse, a medical assistant, and a clerical assistant who provide continuous comprehensive care and whom the patient comes to know and trust. This system has been endorsed by the largest primary care organizations in the U.S. and is emerging as the model of care for Veterans Administration ambulatory clinics.

Application of Rule 3: Support Interprofessional Collaboration

Organizations that value relationships among colleagues design care delivery to support interprofessional collaboration. When teamwork and effective communication are visible and relationships are consistent, patients feel safe and held. When the team is disconnected, the patient's anxiety soars (Koloroutis & Trout, 2012).

Though the concepts of collaboration and coordination are related, there are differences. Coordination entails bringing separate pieces of care into a coherent whole, while collaboration refers to the interactions of people. Interprofessional collaboration increases the likelihood of a higher level of quality and safety than would be possible if the same individual professionals were working separately. You could say that coordination requires reaching out horizontally to bring people and pieces together, while collaboration asks people to dive more deeply into partnership and consultation before action is taken.

Ideally, collaboration leads to a whole that is greater than the sum of the parts. It involves interpersonal skills, including listening and compromise. Earlier in this chapter, we cited Steve Jobs' cancer treatment as an example of absent care coordination. It is a reasonable guess that collaboration in his case was also not optimal. Time and space are needed to develop relationships. This must be understood and considered morally valuable.

Application of Rule 3: Treat the Electronic Health Record (EHR) as Your Electronic Team Member

The EHR is a powerful tool for collaboration and communication. It creates a shared repository of information that is available wherever and whenever it is required. For patients with many comorbidities, it may be *only* the EHR that holds the entire picture. The primary care clinic team at Park Nicollet's Smart Care Clinic in Minneapolis embraces the EHR as the one member of the team that always holds information about the patient. "The EHR is a challenging but necessary part of the care team," we were told by physician Kris Kopski, "It may not have been our choice, but we're in a relationship with the EHR, and we're not only dedicated to making it work; we're dedicated to having the healthiest, most productive relationship possible with our electronic team member."

The need for a healthy, productive relationship with the EHR is particularly strong in integrated delivery systems where the EHR spans hospitals, primary care clinics, specialty clinics, home care, hospice, pharmacies, and

Time and space are needed to develop relationships. This must be understood and considered morally valuable.

sometimes even nursing homes. Modern EHRs are far from perfect, and many people chafe under how their addition has changed their workflow; however, the EHR is here to stay. Thus, your organization's narrative around the EHR influences your care delivery design and the utility of the EHR itself. Does your narrative deem the EHR to be an oppressor victimizing team members? If so, your system design will struggle with reaping its potential benefits, and its value will be limited. In contrast, if your cultural narrative around the EHR is similar to that of the Park

Nicollet Smart Care Clinic, your road to successfully integrating the EHR into the culture of your organization could even be pleasurable.

Leadership for Relationship-Based Care Delivery Design

If an organization's care delivery is to be exemplary, leaders at all levels must consistently model the three simple rules of care delivery design—hold the patient and family, make the best way the easiest way, and support all relationships. This begins with understanding that the attributes of a system emerge from the interaction of people, processes, and structures. This means that when care delivery design is found lacking, the leader does not begin with blaming people, but rather displays curiosity and wonder about the entire system. Leadership by attuning and wondering is a good way to embed the three rules. Leaders invite patients and families into their meetings and ask teams how they have included patients in their improvement efforts. Leaders invite teams to wonder about whether they have made the best way the easiest way and have minimized reliance on memory. Leaders encourage teams to think about the quality of their relationships with one another, with patients and families, and with themselves.

Health care leaders frequently receive letters complaining about care. These letters offer opportunities to model the rules for advancing care delivery design that is relationship-based. A patient complaint is an expression of pain and suffering. When a patient takes the risk (and it does feel risky) to communicate dissatisfaction with the very people who may hold his life in their hands, the work of the leader is to become interested—even fascinated—by the information, by the expressed vulnerability of the person, and by the unique opportunity to gain understanding and improve care. They humble us and challenge us by providing unique opportunities for important growth. The leader thus models being fascinated rather than burdened, respectful of the courage it took for the patient to step forward, appreciative of the patient's willingness to teach us about his experience, and eager to learn and apply what we learn. It's a delicate balance for leaders to hold patients and families, modeling what it means to wonder, while clearly holding the members of the health care team at the same time. Unless staff members feel safe and held during the process, it shuts down their capacity to wonder, and defensiveness will derail the inquiry.

Leaders must also continuously communicate that the organization is involved in a noble cause and that we will never let ourselves be less than the best we can be. To that end, the leader embraces continuous improvement at all levels of the organization. Any effective system of patient care delivery must have organized structures for continuously measuring, challenging, and improving its processes. The organization must also recognize the potential for change fatigue. Changing complex systems is difficult, nonlinear, and unpredictable. Prodigious efforts may result in no discernable improvements. Conversely, tiny changes may result in enormous changes in the system, for better or for worse. For those reasons and more, improving care delivery must be approached with humility. Continuous measurement is necessary to determine whether change has resulted in improvement that outweighs undesirable unintended consequences. Different methodologies (LEAN, Appreciative Inquiry, PDSA, Six Sigma, Root Cause Analysis, etc.) can be employed depending on the issue and the improvement process chosen by the organizations.

Improving care delivery must be approached with humility.

Above all, leaders advancing relationship-based care delivery design must model care and compassion in all of their relationships, expect others to do the same, and embed the four relational practices within organizational processes. Attuning, wondering, following, and holding improve all relationships. The use of these practices is an ideal expression of reverence for the complexity and sacredness of the work. As a leader improves all of her relationships, there is a ripple effect as an increased spirit of partnership pervades the organization. As any team sets out to design its care delivery system, the team must be as relationally proficient as it is technically proficient. That combination alone positions your organization to create a care delivery system in which patients and families are held, all processes are safe and efficient, and everyone in the organization feels valued.

Summary of Key Thoughts

- Good care delivery design results in care that is the safest possible with the best possible outcomes, while patients and families experience being held in the center. Poor design causes avoidable human suffering, poor outcomes, and unnecessary deaths.

- People designing care delivery have an obligation to become students of the experience of illness and physical and emotional trauma. It is essential for designers of care to understand the lived experiences of those receiving care in order to design effective systems.

- Complex adaptive systems, such as care delivery systems, can be viewed as emerging from a handful of simple rules applied over and over. The three rules of care delivery design are:

    1. Hold the patient and family.

    2. Make the best way the easiest way.

    3. Support all relationships.

- Rule 1—Hold the patient and family—means that we cannot presume to know what is best without actively seeking the patient's and family's perspective. This means involving them along the entire design process, including evaluating the current system, prioritizing improvements, designing changes, evaluating success, and planning further refinements.

- Rule 2—Make the best way the easiest way—compels us to design systems that minimize reliance on human memory in order to free up the cognition of clinicians for judgment and critical thinking skills. It also compels us to improve care coordination and support continuity of clinicians.

- Rule 3—Support all relationships—is actualized through processes and structures that promote continuity of clinician-patient relationships and interprofessional collaboration. This sets the stage for knowing the patient as a person.

- Care delivery design is most successful when the people closest to the work are involved in creating and revising their own systems, because no one knows the work better; if people are engaged in innovating the design, they will feel more ownership for the work and want to participate in subsequent improvements.

- Health care professionals have an obligation to attune, wonder, follow, and hold with patients, families, and colleagues. Organizations have an obligation to design systems that actively promote these practices.

- When teams are not functioning in the ways they are intended to function, it may be that someone has been asked to take responsibility and full accountability, but has not been given the authority necessary to achieve what he has taken responsibility for.

- When patients have complaints about their care, the work of the leader is to become interested—even fascinated—by the information and by the unique opportunity they provide for us to gain understanding and improve care. It's vital for leaders to hold staff members throughout these explorations so that they can feel safe enough to retain their ability to wonder and solve problems.

- When leaders are focused on continual improvement of care delivery, they signal that the organization is involved in a noble cause and that we will never let ourselves be less than the best we can be.

Reflection

- In what ways does your organization do an exemplary job of holding the patient and family? What is one way in which you could improve?

- What is your organization currently doing to ensure that the voices of the patient and family are present in your care delivery discussions and design? What more could you do to ensure that all of your systems, processes, and structures help patients and families feel held?

- In your organization, are patient concerns generally seen as welcome information for improvement or as a troublesome problem to be fixed? Discuss the implications of both positions.

- Why would it matter to patients and families that members of the care team have healthy relationships with each other? Why would it matter that people who don't work closely with patients (for example, an HR manager and a person working in housekeeping) still have healthy relationships with each other?

SECTION FIVE
Evidence

CHAPTER ELEVEN
Evidence that Relationship-Based Cultures
Improve Outcomes

CHAPTER TWELVE
Relationship-Based Care and Magnet® Designation

That some achieve great success,
is proof to all that others can achieve it as well.

ABRAHAM LINCOLN

CHAPTER ELEVEN

Evidence that Relationship-Based Cultures Improve Outcomes

ANN FLANAGAN PETRY, SUSAN WESSEL, AND CATHERINE PERRIZO

When everyone in health care has a shared goal of holding patients at the center of care and focusing on the three key relationships (relationship with self, co-workers, and patients and families), outcomes are positively impacted. There is compelling research demonstrating correlations between cultures in which relational competence is normative, and improvement in several areas:

1. Quality, safety, and patient experience

2. Employee and physician engagement

3. Financial health

In this chapter, we will present systematic reviews, meta-analyses, and contemporary studies summarizing evidence of the role relational competence plays in improving organizational cultures and outcomes. We will use current studies from the literature to illuminate how healthy relationships improve health care practices and provide evidence of the efficacy of the formal model known as Relationship-Based Care (RBC).

Peer-Reviewed Studies on the Impact of Relational Competence on Quality, Safety, and Patient Experience

A Nonpunitive (Relational) Approach to Errors Improves Safety

The impact of organizational culture is a recurrent theme in patient safety and quality research. A pioneer in patient safety, Dr. Lucien Leape, declared in testimony before a U.S. Senate committee, "The single greatest impediment to error prevention in the medical industry is that we punish people for making mistakes" (*Patient Safety*, 2001). In fact, traditionally in health care, failure has been punished. Consequently, people may conceal errors and refuse to acknowledge that problems exist (Nieva & Sorra, 2003). An alternative to a punitive philosophy is the Just Culture model, widely used in the aviation industry (GAIN, 2004; Reason, 1998). A key ingredient of Just Culture is the development of organization-wide trust, which, as we know, is built

For a Just Culture to flourish, people must feel protected and held when they report errors and near misses.

through application of the relational practices of attuning, wondering, following, and holding. For a Just Culture to flourish, people must feel protected and held when they report errors and near misses. A Just Culture recognizes that human error is inevitable and that most errors are the result of system breakdown, not bad people, and sees near misses and errors as opportunities to improve. Opportunities for learning are lost when people feel they will be punished or judged harshly. In fact, the essence of patient safety and Just Culture is a supportive environment of *shared* accountability in which candid communication and organizational learning are valued.

In 2004, the U.S. Department of Health and Human Services Agency for Healthcare Research and Quality (AHRQ) began offering the Hospital Survey on Patient Safety Culture. The AHRQ staff survey and comparative database is designed to help hospitals assess their culture of safety. The 2016 findings from 680 hospitals and nearly half a million hospital staff members indicate that hospitals with stronger safety cultures—those in which teamwork was rated as healthy, shame and blame were not evident, fatigue and stress were relatively low, and people felt they had the resources necessary to treat patients safely—had better scores on Patient Safety Indicators (PSIs). PSIs help hospitals and health care organizations assess, monitor, track, and improve the safety of inpatient care (AHRQ, 2016). Per millions of data points, hospitals with better scores on safety climate dimensions also had fewer safety problems.

The organizational change with the most potential for improvement involves nonpunitive response to error—in other words, advancing environments in which staff feel safe to openly discuss errors or near misses without feeling shamed. Other opportunities include promoting relational competence around patient care transitions in which team members share information and hold the patient through transfers to different units or to outpatient settings.

Strong Therapeutic Relationships Improve Health Outcomes

Numerous studies confirm that a strong therapeutic relationship between clinician and patient is fundamental to safe, high-quality care. In a landmark meta-analysis of 127 academic studies, Zolnierek and DiMatteo found that there was a 19% higher risk of nonadherence among patients whose physicians communicated poorly than among patients whose physicians communicated well. These authors concluded that educating physicians in communication skills resulted in significant improvements in patient adherence to treatment. When a physician is trained in communication, the odds of patient adherence to the treatment plan are 1.62 times higher than when a physician receives no training (Zolnierek & DiMatteo, 2009).

Additional reviews of the literature have addressed the significance of relational factors in health outcomes as well. A large systematic review of academic literature found that physicians who adopt a warm, friendly, and reassuring manner are more effective than those who keep consultations formal and do not offer reassurance (Di Blasi, Harkness, Ernst, Georgiou, & Kleijnen, 2001; Griffin et al., 2004; Mumford, Schlesinger, & Glass, 1982; Ong, de Haes, Hoos, & Lammes, 1995; Stewart, 1995; Stewart et al., 2000).

Relational Competence within Teams is Key to Safety and Overall Quality

Observational studies found only weak to moderate associations between ratings of teamwork skills and measures of technical performance. In contrast, in a study of surgeons, analyses of adverse events in surgery revealed that many underlying causes are *behavioral* (such as communication failure) rather than technical (Yule et al., 2006). The authors noted that nontechnical skills such as interpersonal (i.e., relational) skills are not addressed explicitly in surgical training (Gittell, 2009; Gittell, 2016; Moorthy et al., 2005; Yule et al., 2006). Additionally, although patient handoffs have been extensively studied, they are still an area that most health care systems can target for improvement in quality and safety. Poor handoffs characterized by miscommunication and lack of collaboration are associated with increased costs and the quality and safety factors of morbidity and

In a study of surgeons, analyses of adverse events in surgery revealed that many underlying causes are behavioral (such as communication failure) rather than technical.

mortality (Edmundson, 2012; Gittell, 2016). Interestingly, research confirms that hospitals should prioritize teamwork across units and strive to improve meaningful communication across the organization or system in efforts to improve quality and safety during patient transitions (Richter, McAlearney, & Pennell, 2016).

Empirical evidence also supports the need for system improvements such as formal practices to strengthen communication and relationships among interprofessional teams. For example, daily multidisciplinary rounds shorten length of stay for trauma patients (Dutton et al., 2003). Specific communication practices such as team briefings, safety huddles, and safety pauses immediately before surgery have proven effective (Manser, 2009), demonstrating that improvements in relational competence advance both quality and safety.

Healthy Work Environments Reduce Patient Mortality and Morbidity

Hospitals with well-staffed, high-quality nursing environments were found to have fewer patient deaths after surgery than hospitals without those environments (Silber, Rosenbaum, McHugh, Ludwig, & et al., 2016). These researchers matched 25,752 surgical patients at 35 hospitals with "good nursing environments" (all 35 were Magnet-designated hospitals with overall staffing that included more than one RN for every hospital bed) to 25,752 similarly-aged and equally ill patients at 293 hospitals without those nursing environments, and found that the hospitals with better nursing environments had lower post-operative mortality rates and fewer complications for about the same cost. Similarly, Aiken and colleagues' research in the U.S. showed that investments in "better nurse staffing" improved patient outcomes *only* if hospitals also had good work environments. Best practices such as those assessed for Magnet recognition are being implemented across the health care industry (Aiken et al., 2011; Kelly, McHugh, & Aiken, 2011).

Research found that lower patient mortality after acute myocardial infarction was more closely correlated with a positive organizational culture than with whether the organizations used evidence-based treatment protocols.

Similarly, research led by the Yale School of Public Health involving multiple organizations found that lower patient mortality after acute myocardial infarction was more closely correlated with a positive organizational culture than with whether the organizations used evidence-based treatment protocols. The cultural aspects associated with highest survival included unified values and goals, a culture of learning, open communication and collaboration, and involvement by senior leadership (Curry et al., 2011).

Clinicians' Relational Competence Improves Adherence to Treatment Plan, Patient Satisfaction, and Overall Health Status

A study of 7,200 adults by Safran and colleagues explored the impact of physicians' verbal and nonverbal communication on the patient experience and patients' adherence to treatment. Trust in their physicians was the variable most strongly associated with patients' satisfaction with their physicians. Indeed, "patients' trust in their physician" and "physicians' knowledge of patients" are leading correlates of three important outcomes of care: (1) adherence to physician's advice, (2) patient satisfaction, and (3) improved health status (Safran et al., 1998).

Using data from more than 3,000 U.S. acute care hospitals, Press Ganey (2013) conducted an analysis of the eight Hospital Consumer Assessment of Healthcare Providers and Systems (HCAHPS) dimensions describing the patient experience. Press Ganey's analysis identified five HCAHPS dimensions that consistently cluster together:

- Communication with nurses

- Responsiveness of hospital staff

- Pain management

- Communication about medication

- Overall hospital experience rating

Most importantly, higher scores on "communication with nurses"—an indication of nurses' relational competence—correlates with higher scores on the other four measures. This means that when hospitals seek to improve overall, the most influential measure to improve is nurse communication. The implication is also clear that when nurses (and all staff) listen and attune to patients and families, health care systems will likely see gains in other major areas, including Overall Rating. The study was completed using data from 3,062 U.S. acute care hospitals in the CMS Hospital Compare Database (Press Ganey Associates, Inc., 2013).

When hospitals seek to improve overall, the most influential measure to improve is nurse communication.

All Five Drivers of Exceptional Patient/Family Experience Require Relational Competence

Increasingly, measurement of patients' experience is an important factor in assessing overall performance. For example, the Institute for Healthcare Improvement (IHI, 2016) conducted an in-depth analysis of exemplar organizations to reveal specific behaviors or drivers of exceptional patient and family hospital experience. Figure 11.1 depicts the five primary drivers of exceptional care identified by these authors. Note that relational competence is critical to each of these drivers.

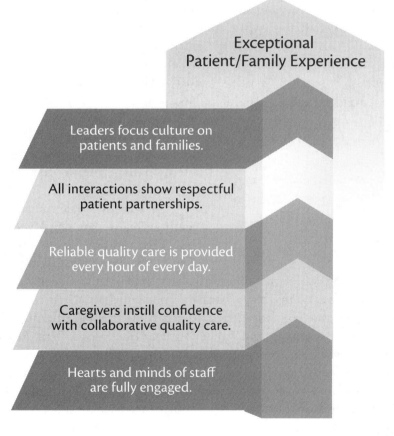

Figure 11.1: Five Primary Drivers of Exceptional Patient/Family Experience

Peer-Reviewed Studies of the Impact of Relational Competence on Employee and Physician Engagement

Relational Competence Positively Impacts Employee Engagement

Positive workplace relationships are foundational to employee engagement and retention. In fact, two of the top five drivers of employee satisfaction—relationships with co-workers and relationships with direct managers—are critical to employee engagement and retention (Caldwell, 2011; Finn & Donovan, 2013). Relationship skill building focused on compassion, integrity, trust, and optimism is vital, as these behaviors have been shown to foster an increase in meaning, high-quality connections, and wellbeing, while simultaneously buffering against stress, burnout, fatigue, and depression (Cameron, 2003; Worline & Dutton, 2017). Health care organizations have an opportunity to explicitly address the importance of positive workplace relationships via practices such as group reflection and intentionally bringing people with diverse talents together, highlighting the shared noble purpose of healing. Health care employees find that reconnecting with meaning at work by explicitly talking about and cultivating compassion, integrity, trust, and optimism leads to higher-quality connections with patients and colleagues, along with increased coordination and collaboration across care settings (Cameron, 2003). Additionally, Bachmann and Zaheer, in their *Handbook of Trust Research* (2006), emphasize that the importance of trust within organizations cannot be overstated. Studies show that the level of trust between managers and staff, within and among teams, and even trust in the institution itself, impacts nearly every business performance metric, including patient loyalty, patient safety, and quality of care (Bartkus & Davis, 2000; Druskat & Wolff, 2001; Duhigg, 2016; Edmundson, 2012).

Health care employees find that reconnecting with meaning at work by explicitly talking about and cultivating compassion, integrity, trust, and optimism leads to higher-quality connections with patients and colleagues, along with increased coordination and collaboration across care settings.

Evidence of the Effectiveness of Emotional and Social Intelligence is Evidence of the Value of Relational Competence

Discovering *why* relational aspects of health care delivery are so important to quality and safety rests in understanding the pivotal role that emotional and social intelligence play. Daniel Goleman defines emotional intelligence as the capacity to recognize one's own and other people's emotions and to use this knowledge to guide thinking and behavior (1998). He defines social intelligence as the ability to successfully navigate complex relationships and environments. Numerous studies demonstrate the impact of emotional intelligence in the workplace. Based on studies of tens of thousands of people in diverse settings, we know that technical knowledge and functional competence are vitally important, yet there is copious evidence that competence in emotional and social intelligence, which contribute in clear ways to relational competence, is the differentiating factor between great and average employees and leaders (Akerjordet & Severinsson, 2007; Boyatzis, Goleman, & McKee, 2002; Cherniss & Goleman, 2001; Goleman, 1998; McQueen, 2003).

> *Competence in emotional and social intelligence, which contribute in clear ways to relational competence, is the differentiating factor between great and average employees and leaders.*

Education in emotional intelligence and communication skills—education designed to improve relational competence—has been shown to positively impact physician-patient relationships and to support empathetic interactions, high-quality teamwork, effective communication, stress management, organizational engagement, physician and nurse career satisfaction, and effective leadership. Several dozen nursing research studies also demonstrate a correlation between emotional intelligence and nurse performance, retention, stress adaptation, organizational citizenship, and selected positive patient clinical outcomes (Amendolair, 2003; Birks & Watt, 2007; Cadman & Brewer, 2001; Elam, 2000; Epstein & Hundert, 2002).

Relational Competence Positively Impacts Physician Engagement

Burnout is prevalent among U.S. physicians, more so than among other U.S. workers, and research suggests that primary care physicians are at greater risk than physicians in other specialties (Shanafelt, 2009). There is overwhelming evidence that burnout adversely affects quality of care as well as physician health. Research indicates that supportive relations, which include positive personal relationships, effective professional relationships, and good communication all serve as important mechanisms for building physician resilience (Jensen, Trollope-Kumar, Waters, & Everson, 2008). Additional studies show the importance of finding meaning in work; principally, meaningful connection with patients and families serves to reduce burnout (Shanafelt, 2009).

Peer-Reviewed Studies of the Impact of Relational Competence on Financial Performance

Relational Competence Improves HCAHPS Scores, and Thus Reimbursement

Research confirms that higher scores on HCAHPS questions including relational measures such as "nurses listening" and "doctors explaining information" correlate with decreased readmissions, thus avoiding the financial penalties connected with readmission within 30 days (Hachem et al., 2014). Further, to investigate the opportunity for hospitals to achieve better care at lower cost, researchers looked at six years of data from nearly 3,000 acute care hospitals. Their analysis revealed that good communication between caregivers and patients has the largest impact on reducing costly readmissions. In fact, the results indicated that a hospital would, on average, reduce its readmission rate by 5% if it were to prioritize communication with patients in addition to complying with evidence-based standards of care (Senot, Chandrasekaran, & Ward, 2015).

Relational Competence Decreases Adverse Outcomes and Malpractice Claims

In a review of 54 malpractice incidents in an emergency department, a devastating 8 of 12 deaths were judged to have been preventable if appropriate teamwork had occurred (Risser et al., 1999). The prevalence of teamwork failures has been attributed to several factors. The professional hierarchy in medicine can inhibit teamwork because first-line staff may not feel that it is safe or normative to speak up (Nembard & Edmondson, 2006). Additionally, research by The Schwartz Center for Compassionate Healthcare has documented that compassionate, patient-centered communication and care are associated with fewer malpractice claims and reduced health care expenditures, among other outcome metrics (Levinson, Roter, Mullooly, Dull, & Frankel, 1997; The Schwartz Center, 2015).

> *Compassionate, patient-centered communication and care are associated with fewer malpractice claims and reduced health care expenditures.*

Cultures in which "Companionate Love" is Normative Improve their Financial Performance

Often the most readily measured financial impacts in health care environments are turnover and staff retention costs. But in a 16-month longitudinal study at a long-term health care facility involving 185 employees, 108 patients, and 42 of those patients' family members, Barsade and O'Neill measured the effect of what they termed *companionate love* on emotional and behavioral outcomes of employees, as well as on health outcomes of patients and the satisfaction of those patients' family members. Companionate love can best be described as showing compassion, caring, and kindness to others (Barsade & O'Neill, 2014).

To conduct their research, Barsade and O'Neill constructed a scale designed to measure tenderness, compassion, affection, and caring. But rather than simply asking the participants if they felt or expressed those emotions themselves, the researchers asked to what degree people saw their colleagues expressing them. They also brought in independent raters to observe the facility's culture and asked family members to rate the culture. Lastly, they added ratings of "cultural artifacts" (how the culture is displayed in the physical environment) that reflect a culture of companionate love—for example, having spaces with a "homey" environment, throwing birthday parties, etc.

One of the most significant findings in the study was that a culture of companionate love reduces employees' withdrawal from work, a key financial drain on health care organizations. Barsade and O'Neill measured employee withdrawal by surveying workers about their levels of emotional exhaustion and by studying their rates of absenteeism. They found that units with higher levels of companionate love had lower levels of absenteeism and employee withdrawal. The researchers also discovered that a culture of companionate love led to higher levels of employee engagement with their work via improved teamwork and employee satisfaction. Not surprisingly, the study also found that the culture of companionate love rippled out from staff members to influence patients and their families. "Certified nursing assistants rated the mood of the residents, and the outside observers rated the culture. Those outside observers could predict that [patients] would be in a better mood if the culture among the staff was more loving," Barsade says (Wharton University of Pennsylvania, 2014).

Findings on the Impact of Relationship-Based Care on Organizations

Relationship-Based Care (RBC) was developed on the evidence-based premise that the quality of three key relationships—relationship with self, with colleagues, and with patients and their families—will determine a great deal about the culture of an organization or work area. When these relationships are healthy, a culture of caring is created in which patients and families feel safe, held with regard, and listened to, all of which contribute to their receiving the highest-quality care. Further, employees in RBC organizations feel empowered and trusted (because they are) and therefore engaged and satisfied. The RBC model (Figure 11.2) and the supporting programs for implementation integrate eight dimensions that support high quality clinical caregiving. These eight dimensions are Healing Culture, Patient and Family (in the center of care), Leadership, Teamwork, Interprofessional Practice, Care Delivery, System Design, and Evidence. RBC advances cultures in which relational competence is normative.

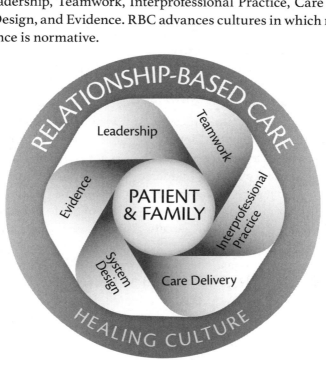

Figure 11.2: Dimensions of Relationship-Based Care

Use of RBC has been proven to positively impact the following outcomes:

1. Patient safety, quality, and experience

2. Employee engagement and satisfaction

3. Financial performance

We will share some examples of outcomes that health care organizations have published or provided to us. See Appendix D for additional outcomes reported by RBC organizations.

RBC Positively Impacts Patient Safety, Quality, and Experience

Lucile Packard Children's Hospital at Stanford in Palo Alto, California selected Relationship-Based Care as its care delivery model after reviewing research demonstrating a relationship between better care environments and better patient outcomes. Hedges and colleagues noted in their published findings, "When optimized, [RBC] can result in safe, patient-centered, well-communicated, and well-coordinated care." One change project the staff in the maternity unit implemented as part of RBC was standardized patient handoffs. They reported their findings from this new standardized patient handoff system: "79% of nurses receiving patients reported feeling better prepared to assume responsibility for the patients' care. Although no pre-implementation patient safety data related to RN handoffs were available, perceived improvements in patient safety because of the handoff process were striking: 68% of nurses reported that omissions, errors, duplications, or near misses were identified during the handoff process. Nurses described 30 patient safety-related issues, nearly 50% of which were medication-related, including documentation errors and verification issues. Catching missed laboratory orders in the EHR resulted in early interventions and aborted care failures" (Hedges, Nichols, & Filoteo, 2012).

Other impacts on patient safety and quality at Lucile Packard include reductions in falls, central line infections, and ventilator-associated pneumonia. Improved response to call lights is another frequent finding. (See Appendix E for more outcomes achieved by organizations using RBC.)

RBC Positively Impacts Employee Engagement and Satisfaction

A Surgical Medical Care Center at Deaconess Hospital in Evansville, Indiana implemented Relationship-Based Care as part of an initiative to use evidence-based changes to improve patient care and job satisfaction. One focus of the initiative was increasing HCAHPS scores. At the initiation of their RBC implementation, the Center's HCAHPS scores were mixed. Patients indicated that 75% of the time "nurses treated me with courtesy and respect," and 50% of the time patients agreed that "nurses listened to me carefully." In addition, 50% of the time patients agreed that "nurses explained in a way I understand," and 58% of the time they indicated that "communication with nurses" was good. After two years, HCAHPS scores had increased to 100% of the time in the category "nurses treated me with courtesy and respect"; 86% of the time "nurses listened to me carefully"; 86% of the time "nurses explained in a way I understand"; and 90% of the time "communication with nurses" was good (Woolley et al., 2012).

Since incorporating *See Me as a Person* workshops as part of Relationship-Based Care, Pennsylvania Hospital in Philadelphia reported percentile changes in the following patient experience questions:

- "Communication with nurses" improved by 34%.

- "Nurses treat with courtesy/respect" improved by 42%.

- "Nurses listen carefully to you" improved by 50%.

- "Nurses explain in a way you understand" improved by 11%.

Chief nurse executive Mary Del Guidice stated, "Patient satisfaction was our Achilles' heel in this organization ... Since we've incorporated *See Me as a Person* education, we've moved consistently from single digit percentile rankings to the 71st percentile last quarter" (Personal communication, January 21, 2016).

Georgia Persky, former chief nurse executive at New York Presbyterian, The University Hospital of Columbia and Cornell in New York City, led a multi-year implementation of RBC, including its care delivery system, Primary Nursing. She partnered with researcher John Nelson to study the impact of RBC on patient satisfaction and the health care work environment for employees. Persky reported that over five years, the Press Ganey overall raw score for patient experience improved between two and six points in every area, which is a significant increase. While all five facilities in that system focused on initiatives to put patients first, only Persky's efforts using RBC resulted in significant improvement in patient satisfaction (Persky, Felgen, & Nelson, 2012). Persky further notes, "Clearly RBC has had a major impact on organizational climate, professional culture, and caring among caregivers for themselves, their colleagues, and their patients" (p. 139). Additionally, Persky reported reductions in voluntary turnover, increased caregiver satisfaction, and reduced rates of falls and infections associated with implementation of RBC (Persky, 2013).

Relationship-Based Care strongly impacts the work environment for staff, as well as their level of engagement. Shared governance and staff empowerment are key tenets of RBC. "Staff engagement and first-line empowerment practices are cited as factors that promote the ability and motivation of frontline staff to improve the quality of care" (Wessel, 2012, p. 188). These concepts are foundational to shared governance and staff empowerment. "A Chicago hospital implementing RBC in all of its nursing departments . . . achieved nurse job enjoyment scores significantly above the average for Magnet hospitals . . . A Dallas facility showed progressive increases in employee engagement, physician satisfaction, and top box patient experience scores over 3 years" (Wessel, 2016, pp. 18-19).

RBC Positively Impacts Organizations' Financial Health

Crittenton Hospital Medical Center, a 290-bed acute care facility located in Rochester, Michigan, realized significant cost savings due to RBC. Before they implemented RBC, overall patient satisfaction scores were at a devastating 7th percentile, and nurse turnover was 18%. Three years into their RBC journey, patient satisfaction was at the 83rd percentile, with one quarterly measure as high as the 99th percentile. During that time, nurse turnover dropped to 3% and there was a waiting list of nurses who wanted to join the organization (Creative Health Care Management, 2010). Spending on agency nurses also decreased significantly. In fact, after spending nearly $2,000,000 per year prior to RBC, within 18 months Crittenton Hospital Medical Center had eliminated agency nursing completely (Van Wagoner, 2013).

St. Mary's Medical Center in Evansville, Indiana selected Relationship-Based Care as its model for achieving Magnet designation. They noted that RBC aligned with the hospital's mission, vision, and values. One outcome they realized from implementing RBC was a significant decrease in nurse turnover. They reported, "Prior to RBC implementation, nurse turnover was 9.4%. Turnover decreased to 8.7% during the RBC training period and decreased to 1.9% at 1 year after implementation" (Winsett & Hauck, 2011, p. 288).

The cost of turnover for an individual nurse varies from $20,000 (Duffield, Roche, Homer, Buchan, & Dimitrelis, 2014) to a range of $42,000 to $64,000, depending on specialty area, because of costs of orientation and lost productivity (Drenkard, 2010). There are multiple benefits of nurse retention, including "reduction in recruitment costs, reduction in orientation costs, productivity gains, decreased patient errors and improved quality of care, increased levels of trust and accountability, and deep organizational knowledge" (Drenkard, 2010, p. 266).

Mississippi Baptist Medical Center in Jackson, Mississippi, reported significant financial impacts at their three-year mark in implementing RBC (Creative Health Care Management, 2014). Chief nurse executive Bobbie Ware describes the decision by executives to implement RBC: "The goal was to see improvement in every measure, but we were committed to doing it with a staff-driven model" (Creative Health Care Management, 2014). After implementation, Ware shared these financial outcomes:

- Reduction in nurse turnover saved $1.6 million annually.

- Elimination of agency staff saved $4.65 million in agency costs.

- Value-based purchasing reimbursement increased more than $250,000.

Implications

We've presented evidence of correlations between relational competence and improvements in quality, safety, and patient experience; employee and physician engagement; and financial health. Given this evidence, those entrusted to advance the effectiveness and viability of health care systems have a new route. While few if any health care organizations have failed outright to value the importance of healthy relationships, relatively few have made the improvement of relationships a key strategy for improving all other measures.

Perhaps until now it has seemed to be too risky a gambit or too soft a pursuit to attempt improvements in such a broad array of measures through the seemingly narrow aim of improving all relationships.

However, it is now clear that in order to achieve excellence in all of these important outcomes, leaders must advance relationship-based cultures. As it turns out, the yellow brick road of health care leads us "home"— back to the basics, back to what we've known all along: In a business that boils down to "people taking care of people," where care is taken to help people thrive, organizations thrive as well. When people are given the tools and empowerment to take excellent care of themselves, one another, and the patients and families in their care, the overall performance of the organization improves.

In a business that boils down to "people taking care of people," where care is taken to help people thrive, organizations thrive as well.

Summary of Key Thoughts

- Research demonstrates correlations between relational competence and improvement in quality, safety, and patient experience; employee and physician engagement; and financial health.

- A strong therapeutic relationship between clinician and patient is fundamental to safe, high-quality care.

- Research confirms that hospitals should prioritize teamwork across units and strive to improve meaningful communication across the organization or system in efforts to improve quality and safety during patient transitions.

- Research led by the Yale School of Public Health involving multiple organizations found that lower patient mortality after acute myocardial infarction was more closely correlated with a positive culture than with whether the organizations used evidence-based treatment protocols.

- According to research from the Institute for Healthcare Improvement, there are five primary drivers of exceptional care:

    1. Leaders focus culture on patients and families.

2. Hearts and minds of staff are fully engaged.

3. All interactions show respectful patient partnerships.

4. Reliable quality care is provided every hour of every day.

5. Caregivers instill confidence with collaborative quality care.

- Health care employees report that reconnecting with meaning at work by explicitly talking about and cultivating compassion, integrity, trust, and optimism leads to higher-quality connections with patients and colleagues, along with increased coordination and collaboration across care settings.

- A facilitated small-group curriculum for physicians with protected time provided by the institution can improve elements of physician wellbeing, including meaning, empowerment, and engagement in work, and can reduce distress, including depersonalization.

- Good communication between caregivers and patients has the largest impact on reducing readmissions.

- Cultures that support expressions of kindness and compassion experience a reduction in emotional exhaustion and a positive influence on the satisfaction and teamwork of employees.

- Use of the Relationship-Based Care model has been proven to positively impact patient safety, quality, and experience; employee engagement and satisfaction; and financial performance.

Reflection

- What could you start doing today to improve relationships within your organization?

- What evidence indicates that a strong therapeutic relationship between clinician and patient is fundamental to safe, high-quality care?

- What could be done in your organization or work area to help clinicians, administrators, and service people feel more connected to the meaning and purpose of their work?

The secret of joy in work is contained in one word: excellence. To know how to do something well is to enjoy it.

Pearl S. Buck

Chapter Twelve

Relationship-Based Care and Magnet® Recognition

Gen Guanci and Marky Medeiros

The human pursuit of excellence has a tendency to capture our attention. Many of us can name the world's fastest human, and we tend to pay attention, for at least a little while, to whoever wins the Super Bowl, World Series, NBA and WNBA Finals, or World Cup. For the fans, it may be all about their favorite team taking home the prize, but you can bet that for the players, it wasn't all about the final outcome. They pursued excellence, usually from an early age, for one simple reason: They had the *drive* to pursue excellence. They saw potential in themselves, and it's more than likely that someone else, somewhere along their journey, saw potential in them too. We humans pursue excellence because we enjoy the challenge.

In health care, as in sports, we don't pursue a big award for the bragging rights. We pursue the award because of what we know it will do for our organization, our entire staff, and, most importantly, our patients. When an organization pursues a national award or recognition, teams throughout the organization will create, strengthen, and/or deepen structures and processes to meet standards outlined in that award or recognition. In effect, the team is challenged to use innovation, creativity, and

Many health care leaders seek national recognition, not as an end in itself, but as validation of the great work the organization is doing.

out-of-the-box thinking to meet the standards or criteria for even more extraordinary performance.

Many health care leaders seek national recognition, not as an end in itself, but as a specific path to excellence and as validation of the great work the organization is doing. If you have been enjoying good measures of success in your quest to advance a Relationship-Based Care (RBC) culture in your organization, you may also be positioned to begin your official pursuit of national recognition.

Some of the most common award recognition programs for health care organizations include:

- American Association of Critical-Care Nurses Beacon Award for Excellence™ (formerly the Beacon Award)

- Baldrige Performance Excellence Program (formerly the Malcolm Baldrige National Quality Program)

- Best Places to Work

- Great Places to Work©

- Individual state-level quality awards

- Planetree Designation

- The Pinnacle of Excellence Award© (Press Ganey)

- American Nurses Credentialing Center (ANCC) Pathway to Excellence® Program

- American Nurses Credentialing Center (ANCC) Pathway to Excellence in Long Term Care® Program

- American Nurses Credentialing Center (ANCC) Magnet Recognition Program®

While a successful RBC journey positions an organization to pursue any of these awards or recognitions, this chapter will focus on the ways in which RBC and Magnet®* fit together.

Magnet Designation

In the 1980s, during a severe nursing shortage, Margaret McClure, Muriel Poulin, Margaret Sovie, and Mabel Wandelt studied several hospitals throughout the United States that were attracting and retaining nurses despite the dire shortage. The American Nurses Association sponsored this team of researchers to determine what was occurring at those organizations that made them "magnets" for nurses. Their findings, first published in 1983, were grouped into three categories:

1. **Administration:** Flexible work schedules, adequate staffing matrixes, and career growth opportunities

2. **Professional practice:** Professional practice models, nurse autonomy, and a positive image of nursing throughout the organization

3. **Professional development:** Customized orientation plans, support for continuing education, and competency-based clinical advancement programs/clinical ladders

(McClure & Hinshaw, 2002)

In 1993, the American Nurses Credentialing Center (ANCC) established what it then called the Magnet Nursing Services Recognition Program for Excellence in Nursing as a designation that would formally recognize organizations that demonstrated excellence in nursing practice. Since the University of Washington Medical Center in Seattle became the first Magnet®-designated facility in 1994, more than 452 hospitals have received or maintained Magnet status. Fewer than 8% of the

---

* MAGNET®, Magnet Recognition Program®, ANCC®, Magnet®, and the Journey to Magnet Excellence® are registered trademarks of the American Nurses Credentialing Center. The products and services of Creative Health Care Management are neither sponsored nor endorsed by ANCC. All rights reserved.

hospitals in the United States have achieved Magnet status. The full story of how Magnet designation came about can be found in the book *Feel the Pull: Creating a Culture of Nursing Excellence* (Guanci, 2016, pp. 10–18).

While organizations pursuing any national recognition will have an advantage if they are already succeeding in transforming to a relationship-based culture, the alignment between Magnet and Relationship-Based Care (RBC) is particularly significant. The rest of this chapter is an exploration of why it is beneficial to consider a Journey to Magnet Excellence® if RBC is already part of your culture.

How RBC Supports Magnet and Magnet Supports RBC

The Magnet model provides a foundation for us to examine how the five components of Magnet interweave with seven of the dimensions of the RBC model. Figure 12.1 shows the Magnet model.

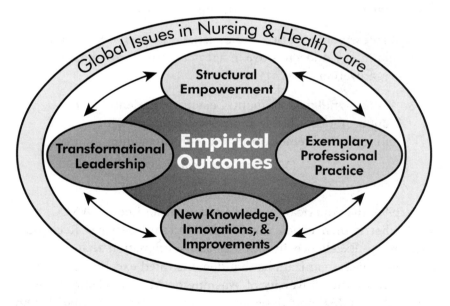

Figure 12.1: The Magnet Model (© 2013 American Nurses Credentialing Center. All rights reserved. Reproduced with the permission of the American Nurses Credentialing Center.)

The five components of the Magnet model are (1) transformational leadership, (2) structural empowerment, (3) exemplary professional practice, (4) new knowledge, innovations, and improvements, and (5) empirical outcomes. Here's how they interweave with seven of the RBC dimensions: patient and family centeredness, leadership, teamwork, interprofessional practice, care delivery, system design, and evidence.

Transformational Leadership in RBC and Magnet

Transformational leadership inspires people at all levels of the organization to join together to advance a common purpose or higher good. The Magnet model component of transformational leadership correlates directly to the RBC dimensions of leadership and of holding the patient and family in the center of our care. The expectations of the Magnet environment include that positional leaders demonstrate the leadership skills of being "knowledgeable risk takers with strong vision" who are "participative, visible, accessible and an advocate of shared decision-making" (ANCC, 2013, p. 20, 24). To satisfy this Magnet requirement:

- RBC supports individual transformational leadership development through self-awareness, commitment to growth, relational competence, and strong collaborative skills (Koloroutis, 2004).

- RBC introduces the Transformational Leadership Cycle, which guides individuals to lead with purpose, inspire a shared vision, and engage in ongoing reflection and courageous risk-taking (Koloroutis, 2004).

- RBC leaders provide the inspiration and infrastructure to support data-driven best practices and staff-driven decisions to strengthen patient care and professional practice (Felgen, 2007).

- RBC introduces the I_2E_2 formula for change as an organizational roadmap that supports transformational change (Felgen, 2007).

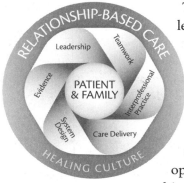

The ultimate purpose of transformational leadership, in pursuit of both Magnet designation and an RBC culture, is to create an environment in which we hold the complex needs of the patient and family in the center of care. Transformational leaders engage their teams in conversations designed to uncover the good they are already doing and point them toward opportunities for enhancements. This is achieved through Appreciative Inquiry methods (Cooperrider & Whitney, 2005), which are embedded in RBC concepts and implementation strategies.

Structural Empowerment in RBC and Magnet

RBC empowers the people closest to the work to design and refine their own systems and processes. This principle is consistent with the structural empowerment component of the Magnet model. Magnet cultures support nurses in having control over the practice environment and assuring that shared decision-making processes are in place. The RBC dimensions of system design and interprofessional practice ensure that RBC implementation is built on a shared decision-making model. RBC educational programs such as *Leading an Empowered Organization* (LEO) educate and support leaders in creating the structural empowerment seen in Magnet environments.

Magnet environments require that the staff voice be evident in personnel policy and procedure development, as well as formal peer feedback at all levels. The leadership dimension of RBC compels leaders to actively support employee engagement through involvement in decision making. Magnet and RBC both view these structural empowerment practices as integral to organizational success.

Exemplary Professional Practice in RBC and Magnet

While Magnet designation was once a recognition given to nursing for extraordinary nursing practice, the Magnet community acknowledges that it takes an entire organization with all professional disciplines working together for quality patient care and superb patient outcomes to happen. Interprofessional team partnerships are now seen as a core element of professional practice.

Magnet cultures support nurses' accountability for the practice environment and coordination of care. RBC helps organizations meet this Magnet requirement because it is built on a theoretical framework that fosters the RN's responsibility, authority, and accountability for patient care decisions.

> *It takes an entire organization with all professional disciplines working together for quality patient care and superb patient outcomes to happen.*

Through the Primary Nurse role, for example, all care is coordinated by a designated RN. In a Magnet environment, autonomous practice and independent judgment are expected of nurses, and this requirement is satisfied through the care delivery dimension of RBC, which facilitates the development of structures and processes that support autonomous patient care decisions by Primary Nurses.

Under this Magnet component, peer support and knowledgeable experts are to be made available to and utilized by the clinical staff. These experts are both internal and external to the organization and are often interprofessional in nature. In RBC, interprofessional peer support is fostered through leadership and council development and involvement, communication processes, and widespread reporting of progress—particularly outcomes.

New Knowledge, Innovations, and Improvements in RBC and Magnet

This Magnet component challenges organizations to seek, conduct, provide, and utilize evidence and research findings in the practice setting. The intention of this dimension is to use new knowledge to enhance outcomes, both for the patient and for the workforce. This correlates with RBC's philosophy that the people closest to the work are in the best position to design and refine their own systems and processes. This Magnet component also correlates specifically with the RBC dimensions of both interprofessional practice and evidence-based practice.

Empirical Outcomes in RBC and Magnet

In Magnet environments, high quality is an organizational priority. This must be confirmed by participation in national databases with demonstrated outcomes that exceed national benchmark means and/or medians. In RBC, outcome measures include patient satisfaction and staff satisfaction and engagement, as well as the quantitative and qualitative data that drive practice changes. In other words, RBC and Magnet (and most other national recognition organizations) want to see high performance in the same three metrics:

1. **Patient outcomes** (e.g., decreases in falls, hospital-acquired infections, hospital-acquired pressure ulcers, and morbidity and mortality)

2. **Employee satisfaction** (e.g., healthy interpersonal work environments, employee safety, perceptions of empowerment, and retention)

3. **Patient satisfaction** (e.g., patients treated with courtesy and respect, involvement of patients in care decisions, responsiveness, pain management, and careful listening)

Magnet Requirement: Creation of a Professional Practice Model

An important aspect of any Magnet journey is the creation of a professional practice model, or PPM. A PPM is a schematic depiction of how nurses in the organization practice, communicate, collaborate, and develop professionally (ANCC, 2013). The presence of a PPM is more than the satisfaction of a Magnet requirement. The thinking that goes into its creation provides a framework for discussing what the entire organization values most.

The key element of a Magnet-required PPM is a care delivery system that is patient- and family-centered. Relationship-Based Care clearly fits that description and has been included in countless PPMs through the years. Figure 12.2 is an example of a PPM that uses RBC as its care delivery system.

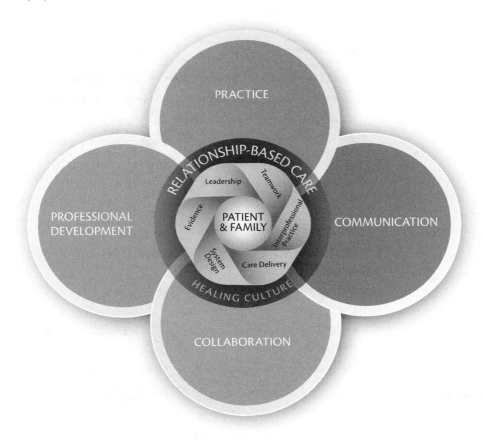

Figure 12.2: A Sample Professional Practice Model Using RBC as Care Delivery System

When you look at the requirements of a PPM through the lens of RBC, it is clear that they are deeply intertwined, which is why so many organizations choose RBC as their care delivery system (Hernandez, 2016; Hozak & Brennan, 2012; Marsh, 2017; York Hospital, 2012). Many organizations that have implemented RBC develop their PPM as an interprofessional model, knowing that it will drive practice in all their clinical and nonclinical disciplines.

Figure 12.3 shows selected features of RBC that support the creation of a PPM that addresses how caregivers practice, collaborate, communicate, and develop professionally.

Magnet PPM Focus	RBC Features and Focus
Practice	Three key relationships (with self, team, and patient and family)
	Four therapeutic practices (attuning, wondering, following, and holding)
	Shared decision-making environment
	Advocates for a council structure for all disciplines and departments
	Driven by evidence-based practice and outcomes
	Built on a theoretical framework
	Reflective practice
Collaboration	Focus on building a culture with a common mission
	Emphasis on relationships with colleagues, including giving and asking for help
	Nursing and interprofessional council structure
	Use of consensus for decision making
	Development of principles of RBC for clinical professional/allied health disciplines
	Development of principles of RBC for support services
Communication	Proactive two-way communication that includes the patient and family and all members of the health care team
	Coordinating council/results council
	Systems to ensure 100% communication to all unit members from and to the unit practice councils
Professional Development	Focus on relationship with self/self-awareness/self-development
	Empowers all employees to leverage their individual talents
	Increased role clarity
	Ongoing education related to RBC implementation and practices
	Ongoing education related to therapeutic relationships
	Ongoing education related to ethics and professional excellence

Figure 12.3: How RBC Supports Creation of a Magnet PPM

Relationship-Based Care clearly supports the components of practice, collaboration, and communication. As for the component of professional development, while RBC establishes a strong developmental foundation and Primary Nursing sets the stage for exemplary professional nursing practice, for those pursuing Magnet designation, the ANCC also looks for additional specific structures and processes related to professional development. Among these are formal peer feedback, competency-based clinical advancement, support for national certification, and BSN completion or higher for all nurses.

While ANCC currently defines only the elements of a *nursing* PPM, nothing prevents organizations from raising the bar and creating a PPM that describes and depicts how all clinical disciplines practice, communicate, collaborate, and develop professionally.

The Necessary Guidance for Success

A Magnet journey is a complex, multiyear process, as are many other recognition awards. In order to be successful, it's important to assess and determine from the outset which internal resources you will use and whether you will use external consultative support. From the beginning, it is important to understand the scope of the designation process and the services that may need to be included for an efficient and successful journey. The services you may need, depending on your organization's starting point, include the following:

- General and/or focused education for a variety of stakeholders

- Coaching and mentoring of the journey leader

- Readiness assessment

- Structure and process development

- Application and support document review and feedback

- Electronic document development

- Site visit preparation

- Year-after support

- Redesignation support (Guanci, 2016)

Before you invest in anything or any*body*, however, we recommend that you form a committee to look into what a Magnet journey entails. A search of articles and books will yield worthwhile information, but nothing is as valuable as talking with others who've been on the journey. If possible, send a group from your organization to the annual ANCC National Magnet Conference®. Every year, upwards of 10,000 people attend the Magnet conference, so it is an excellent opportunity to sit down with people in all phases of the journey to figure out if Magnet is a realistic pursuit for your organization.

The Question of Readiness

If you are implementing RBC and that journey is going well, your organization is likely to have a strong foundation from which to begin a journey to Magnet designation. You already have shared governance, staff councils, department-level and interprofessional councils, leadership support for staff empowerment, as well as outcomes in patient satisfaction, employee satisfaction, and clinical outcomes that exceed (or at least approach) national benchmarks. It is also likely that you have the structures, processes, and outcomes to be successful.

If you are implementing RBC and that journey is going well, your organization is likely to have a strong foundation from which to begin a journey to Magnet designation.

The question of readiness is a pivotal point in shaping the journey toward Magnet designation. A comprehensive readiness assessment defines your current reality and determines what will be required to ultimately submit an application for designation. The assessment identifies gaps in practice and opportunities for improvement—in other words, what is needed to achieve outcomes that outperform national benchmarks. All of these factors determine timing for submitting your application. Assessing where you are and defining where you want to be will determine your unique plan for getting there.

From an organizational culture perspective, embarking on a Magnet journey means that your culture is already striving for excellence, is already excelling in patient outcomes, and is already cultivating an environment in which people want to work. It means your organization already has structures and processes in place that align with the sources of evidence that support excellence. It does not mean your organization is perfect, but it means there is a desire to provide high-quality care in a healthy work environment. Great organizations inevitably strive to be better, so it is not unusual for individuals in these organizations to come together and strengthen areas where there are gaps, build on strengths, and create an experience of common pride. Every step of the journey toward Magnet designation is an opportunity to celebrate accomplishments, cultivate positive energy, and strengthen pride in practice.

Every step of the journey toward Magnet designation is an opportunity to celebrate accomplishments, cultivate positive energy, and strengthen pride in practice.

A readiness assessment identifies your "pure gaps" as well as your opportunities for improvement (OFIs). This is explained in the book *Feel the Pull.*

> The items about which you say, "We don't have that" are referred to as pure gaps. The items about which you say, "We have some, but . . . ," or "We need to improve on . . . ," or "We have this in some areas, but not all . . . ," are opportunities for improvements (OFIs). Regardless of whether you have pure gaps or OFIs, they all need to be addressed. (Guanci, 2016, p. 48)

Becoming clear about your pure gaps and OFIs helps alleviate starts and stops that may occur because the organization prematurely commits to a date for their document submission but then has to change it. This can be dispiriting for everyone involved. That's why it's vitally important for the readiness assessment to be comprehensive, accurate, and objective. A crucial part of the readiness assessment is a clearly outlined "next steps" plan.

A readiness assessment is a comprehensive process that yields some very practical data, as illustrated in Figure 12.4.

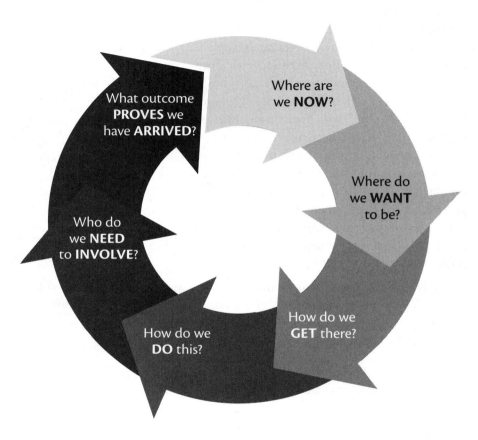

Figure within image: "Where are we **NOW**?", "Where do we **WANT** to be?", "How do we **GET** there?", "How do we **DO** this?", "Who do we **NEED** to **INVOLVE**?", "What outcome **PROVES** we have **ARRIVED**?"

Figure 12.4: Readiness Assessment

Because a thorough and accurate assessment is so important and objective neutrality is critical, an external consultant is often engaged to conduct the **readiness assessment**. This external resource must have thorough knowledge of the specific components of and criteria for Magnet designation and a record of supporting successful designations. This consultant must also be able to generate a comprehensive written report of findings. Many organizations continue to work with the people who conducted their readiness assessment throughout their Magnet journey.

For those organizations that are currently Magnet designated and are moving toward redesignation, a **vulnerabilities assessment** is highly recommended. While similar in approach to a readiness assessment, a vulnerabilities assessment looks at what is different in the designation process since your last designation and what you need to do to ensure that you meet the new standards.

It is our experience that readiness and vulnerabilities assessments are always valuable because they define current reality. Either an organization finds that it is well positioned to pursue initial Magnet designation or redesignation, or it finds out that it has gaps in its culture that it needs to address.

The Benefits of National Recognition

Magnet designation brings significant returns on the organization's investment. Magnet-designated hospitals receive a better bond rating, thereby enabling the organization to procure loans at a lower interest rate. With many of the national recognitions, including Magnet, organizations receive automatic points bestowed by The Leapfrog Group, an organization that promotes improvements in the safety of health care by giving consumers data to make more informed hospital choices. In addition, 80% of the *US News & World Report*'s Top 10 Hospitals (2016), including their top ten for acute care, pediatric, and other specialty organizations, are Magnet-designated.

Magnet designation brings significant returns on the organization's investment.

Another key area of benefit for Magnet organizations is in nurse recruitment and retention. As of April 2017, the average nurse vacancy rate at Magnet hospitals was only 2.31% (ANCC, 2017), with reported national vacancy averages for non-Magnet hospitals in March 2016 standing at 8.5% to 16% depending on the specialty and the region of the country (NSI Nursing Solutions, Inc., 2016).

Beyond any of these very tangible benefits, the advancements to a culture that come with a Magnet journey are nothing short of extraordinary. Organizations on a journey to excellence often say that the journey itself was more meaningful than the actual recognition. Along the journey people come together, learn about the organization, analyze outcomes, make improvements, build relationships, and grow professionally through the process. People at the point of service are working alongside people in formal leadership positions. Roles and titles are forgotten as the team works together to achieve a common goal. A beautiful culture is revealed as the team pulls together. These actions by themselves directly affect employee satisfaction and engagement.

Ask anyone who has been involved in a successful national recognition journey, and you will hear similar themes: "Our journey to excellence was hard work but very rewarding . . . I am so proud of my organization, my department, my unit, and my colleagues . . . This experience restored my passion for my profession . . . It feels wonderful to be recognized for the great work we do every day." Being recognized nationally for the work and outcomes of an organization brings the passion and pride in the organization to a whole new level.

The benefits of Magnet designation include advancing the organization's culture, building pride within your teams, and receiving recognition in the marketplace for the great work being done. There is great satisfaction in receiving the designation that so many people worked so hard to make possible and in knowing that your organization is indeed one of the best of the best.

Being recognized nationally for the work and outcomes of an organization brings the passion and pride in the organization to a whole new level.

Summary of Key Thoughts

- If you've been enjoying good measures of success in your quest to advance a Relationship-Based Care culture in your organization, you may be poised to begin your official pursuit of national recognition.

- Organizations are often successful in their Magnet pursuit due to the strength of their professional practice environment, which includes a strongly encultured care delivery system.

Health care organizations using RBC have a strong foundation on which to build an amazing patient care experience.

- The five components of the Magnet model (transformational leadership; structural empowerment; exemplary professional practice; new knowledge, innovations, and improvements; and empirical outcomes) interweave with seven dimensions of the RBC Model (patient and family centeredness, leadership, teamwork, interprofessional practice, care delivery, systems design, and evidence).

- An important aspect of any Magnet journey is the creation of a professional practice model (PPM). A PPM is a schematic depiction of how professionals practice, communicate, collaborate, and develop professionally.

- A Magnet journey is a complex, multiyear process, as are many other recognition awards. In order to be successful, it's important to assess and determine from the outset how you will use both internal resources and external consultative support.

- The ANCC holds an annual Magnet conference that upwards of 10,000 people attend. This event provides an excellent opportunity to sit down with people in all phases of the journey to figure out whether Magnet is a realistic pursuit for your organization.

- Readiness assessments are always profoundly valuable because they define current reality. Because a thorough and accurate assessment is so important and objective neutrality is critical, an external consultant is often engaged to conduct the readiness assessment.

- Magnet designation brings significant financial returns on the organization's investment, but the financial benefits pale in comparison to the boon that a successful Magnet journey offers an organization's culture and individuals.

Reflection

- Empowerment is an important concept within both the Magnet journey and an RBC culture. Describe ways in which people in your organization are or could be empowered to make decisions affecting their work.

- What do you have in place that supports a national recognition journey?

- What are some of the ways that a Magnet journey and designation could positively affect interprofessional collaboration and employee satisfaction and engagement in your organization?

- What are some ways that a Magnet journey and designation could positively affect clinical outcomes and patient satisfaction in your organization?

The only way the world will change is if many more of us step forward, let go of our judgments, become curious about each other, and take the risk to begin a conversation.

MARGARET WHEATLEY

EPILOGUE

Continuing the Conversation

MARY KOLOROUTIS AND DAVID ABELSON

It is a paradox that our work includes so many painful elements of the human experience and still ends up being, somehow, profoundly beautiful. That contradiction is a lot for any one person to hold. It's even more for a person to effectively make sense of it, to sort it out—to reconcile the paradox of it. Not very many of us can do that kind of reconciling in isolation.

Health care is the work we chose. Why did we choose it? Who are we, that we would run headlong into such work? Most of us even sacrificed a lot to get here—perhaps years of expensive schooling; long, difficult hours; or putting off starting a family. Perhaps it's because we all have a desire to be part of something meaningful, something bigger than ourselves, something that makes a difference, something beautiful.

Could it be that the reason we do this work is not because it is at times uplifting, but instead because it is at times almost impossibly uncomfortable? Is it because of the possibility that we may one day be caring for, all within the span of an hour, the dying 16-year-old victim of a drunk driver, the grieving parent of that dying child, and the drunk driver too? As theologian Henri Nouwen said in his book *In Memoriam*, "Anyone who willingly enters into the pain of a stranger is truly a remarkable person" (1980). It's not so crazy to think that people—not everyone, but some people—would be drawn to work that amplifies all things human. Still, how can you expect to be ready for such things?

We believe the key is conversations. The more we in health care connect with one another about our work, the better we are able to cope when our work puts the unthinkable in our path. Conversations help us transcend our separateness. They give us a forum to think through, feel through, and talk through the sometimes stunning complexities of our work. There is a transmission of sorts that happens among health care people when we connect. We've seen it, but more importantly, we've felt it. In a recent workshop, physician participants were asked to pair with another person in the group and share something going on in their lives or practice that made them feel vulnerable. In debriefing the interaction, a participant said that he had never before been invited to talk about feeling vulnerable. He said that through talking about a situation in which he was privately struggling—and to have someone do nothing more than silently attune, wonder, follow, and hold—he was able to access greater clarity about the situation, and he felt a sense of release from the burden itself. All of this happened within a 5-minute exercise. He said he was struck by how important and helpful this exercise was and that he intended to make such conversations an ongoing part of his practice.

People in all walks of health care are hungry for conversation. Whether our conversations are formal or informal, planned or spontaneous, we find that the more we open ourselves to hearing and speaking the truth of what we experience in our work, the better and more connected we all feel. We share joy over our triumphs, and we cry together over our tragedies. We confess our shortcomings, we ask for help or guidance, we share what we know, and we listen for validation that we are not alone in our uneasiness. For a business in which every experience of every person with every other person is incontestably unique, we have a lot in common.

The patterns of conversation you hear in your organization reveal a lot. In the same way the language a person uses reveals something about the psyche of the person, the conversations that happen within an organization reveal the organization's culture. What do you hear people saying? What would you *like* to hear people saying?

How long has it been since you've paused with intention and really taken in the wonders of health care surrounding you? How long has it been since you took time to marvel at the beauty of the work of human caring and the everyday miracles you get to play a role in every day? This book mentioned several of them—the person who spoke lovingly to a recently deceased man while cleaning the man's body, the person who draped a flag over a deceased veteran to show his own respect and invite the respect of others, the person who told a patient's family member where to find "the good coffee." Because the stakes in our work environments are often so high, everything matters. That's the good news and the bad news, of course. It means that a small, loving gesture can show someone she isn't alone in her pain, restore hope where there was none, and even inspire someone to heal a troubled relationship. It also means that a small act of casual diminishment can cause someone to think that he really is alone in his pain; it can steal hope, or it can provoke tumult in otherwise peaceful relationships.

What is the critical conversation we're not having today that we need to have? Could it be that the most important conversation is the one you don't want to have? We throw ourselves into work that puts difficult situations in front of us every day. So why are we so often reluctant to talk about difficult things? Is it because we know from experience that there is no tidy resolution to be had? When we do talk, it's true that no pat formulas emerge, but we change, we grow, we improve, we feel connected, we feel better.

Early in this book an invitation was issued; you were asked to bring your whole self to your work. As this book ends, we want to issue another invitation: Make time for conversations that matter. Make time for conversations about what it means to be human and vulnerable. Make time to talk about the noble cause of health care and the remarkable people doing this work.

As you finish this book on advancing relationship-based cultures, we hope that you will commit to some concrete actions that will help to advance such a culture in your organization. Advancing a relationship-based culture requires conversation, and we believe that as sacred as the conversations that spring up organically in health care are, structures and processes that invite formal conversations are a necessary part of advancing a culture that is healing for everyone in it.

As a leader or influencer at any level in your organization, you have the power to shift the conversation. If you want to hear more positivity in the cultural narrative, ask people questions about what's working well.

Ask them to tell you about a situation in which they made a positive difference for a patient, family member, or co-worker. Ask them to join you in brainstorming a new vision for an aspect of practice or a structural change that would better support the creation and nurturance of therapeutic relationships. And if you want to hear more depth in the cultural narrative, ask people about how they're coping with the pace or complexity of their work. Ask them whether there is something troubling that you could support them in working through. Ask them about self-care—perhaps about what they have done lately that was really just for them and no one else.

We know that sometimes people are reluctant to have conversations because they can open a Pandora's Box of troubles, grief, or complaints. We may worry that something unexpected will be revealed, and we won't know what to say. You know now, though, that when you attune, wonder, follow, and hold in the face of such things, that is enough—*you* are enough.

It is likely that the pace and complexity of health care are only going to increase. We believe the only thing that will restore the balance in health care is for all of its people to slow down—at least internally, at least for a time—and connect with one another. You have no trouble recognizing that many of your colleagues are extraordinary people, and they have no trouble recognizing the myriad gifts you bring to your work, life, and way of being. When work and life seem to be moving all too quickly, slow down. Connect. Attune, wonder, follow, and hold.

Appendixes

Appendix A
See Me as a Person Therapeutic Practices:
Core Competencies Applied to Pain and Comfort Care

Appendix B
See Me as a Person Therapeutic Practices:
Core Competencies Applied to Teams

Appendix C
Role Clarity Matrix for People-Related Functions

Appendix D
Impact of Relationship-Based Care as Reported by
Organization Leaders

Appendix E
Impact of Relationship-Based Care Found in the Literature

APPENDIX A

See Me as a Person Therapeutic Practices: Core Competencies Applied to Pain and Comfort Care

TARA NICHOLS

This appendix provides a knowledge foundation and explores the requisite clinician mindset and specific application of the therapeutic practices of attuning, wondering, following, and holding to the mission of helping patients move from pain to comfort.

Knowledge and Mindset

Pain is information; it is our body's way of telling us that something is wrong. A pain scale of 0–10 cannot convey this multidimensional signal. In many care settings, however, pain is assessed and treated from a linear/physical perspective, assessing mainly the relative intensity of a somatic sensation (National Pharmaceutical Council, 2001; Pasero & McCaffery, 2011). Patients are often frustrated enough when trying to convey their discomfort with such a limited methodology that they may resort to reporting their pain level as 10 for fear that if they actually rate their physical pain lower, vigilant attempts to identify the source of their discomfort will cease. Conversely, promoting *comfort* evokes hope that someone cares enough to want to relieve suffering, whereas the mention of the word pain may evoke fear (Kolcaba, 2003), including fear that their pain will not be acknowledged, fear that it will not be resolved, or fear that they will be perceived as weak, drug-seeking, and/or needy (Kolcaba, 2003).

It's important to be able to differentiate between addressing an individual's pain and addressing the overall comfort of that individual. According to Kolcaba, comfort is "the immediate state of being strengthened by having the needs for relief, ease, and transcendence addressed in the four contexts of holistic human experience: physical, psychospiritual, sociocultural, and environmental" (1997). Discomfort can be physical, but it can also be mental and/or emotional. Asking only about someone's pain level leaves out anything the person doesn't directly define as pain. When discomforts are not addressed, they have the potential to intensify physical pain and/or lead to unmet basic needs. People can achieve comfort, even within a painful episode; therefore, comfort is more than just the absence of pain.

Every day in systems of care, patients have pain experiences that can include fear, suffering, exclusion from the plan of care, loss of trust in the system of care, severe pain, grief from loss of function, and loss of wellbeing. All these feelings can lead to a state that is worse than the pain itself. Patients may experience overwhelming feelings of powerlessness, isolation, anger, guilt, and vulnerability arising from not being believed and cared for by the people they must rely on. These feelings also inhibit positive modulation of their perception of pain (National Pharmaceutical Council, 2001; Rainville, Bao, & Chretien, 2005; Visser, n.d.).

To provide effective comfort care, clinicians must understand the complexity of pain and discomfort as just described and be aware of the seven conditions that advance comfort, as listed in Figure A.1.

1. **Absence of fear:** feeling relief or the subsiding of emotions of distress aroused by the unknown, the unclear, or perceived harmful and painful experience, real or imagined. State of being: Now that I believe you see me, I feel held and protected; I am at ease.

2. **Trust restored:** feeling the renewed confidence in a person or institution on which one relies. State of being: Now that I believe you see me, I know that you are genuinely interested in me, my values, my beliefs, and our relationship is renewed. You have followed through with your promises.

3. **Absence of pain:** feeling a diminished and/or altered perception of physical suffering and discomfort caused by illness or injury. State of being: Now that I believe you see me, I am in a state of comfort; I am at ease and can focus my energy on coping in this state of vulnerability.

4. **Absence of suffering:** feeling a diminished and/or altered perception of the negative psychological and physiological impact on wellbeing caused by physical pain, disability, or loss that may accompany illness or treatment, including fear, anxiety, confusion, and frustration surrounding the experience of being vulnerable (Dempsey, 2014). State of being: Now that I believe you are my advocate, I choose to partner with you in focusing my being and my energy toward healing.

5. **Sense of wellbeing:** feeling that there is a positive interaction between one's circumstances, activities, and psychological resources—the overall extent and perception of quality of life. State of being: Now that I believe you see me, I am a willing participant in the plan of care and take ownership of the outcomes.

6. **Acceptance of grief/loss of function:** feeling acceptance and understanding concerning one's state as it relates to loss of function. State of being: Now that I believe you see me, and you are not negating the impact of my loss, I can accept the change that it brings.

7. **Perceived inclusion:** feeling connected to care and treatment while in a vulnerable state. State of being: Now that I believe you see me, I am willing to listen to the knowledge you possess to guide my healing. We are connected in a shared vision for my health, and I can rest while I heal.

Figure A.1: The Seven Conditions that Advance Comfort
(Developed by Tara Nichols, MS, RN, CCRN, CCNS, ACNS-BC, AGCNS-BC, and John Nelson, PhD, RN)

Theoretically, when a person perceives a partnership with a caregiver while in a vulnerable state and can believe and trust the caregiver, the individual's capacity to cope, self-soothe, and experience comfort are strengthened. When there is a therapeutic connection, the patient and caregiver are "in it together." The person in our care believes and trusts that we will work with them to maximize their comfort.

When the focus is on comfort, along with pain management, there is a tangible shift away from stigmatizing the patient as "drug-seeking" to seeing the patient as a person seeking relief from pain and hoping to achieve comfort. Behaviors related to the presence of discomfort are often interpreted negatively (e.g., drug-seeking, needy, histrionic, attention-seeking). What if these behaviors were instead interpreted as comfort-seeking behaviors, in which the patient is seen as our chief source of information about what is needed to alleviate pain and suffering? We as humans instinctively seek a comfort experience (Kolcaba, 2003).

Assisting an individual to move from pain to comfort is supported by the use of the four therapeutic practices: attuning, wondering, following, and holding (Koloroutis & Trout, 2012). Tending to a person's comfort needs may alter the prior negative experiences of patients' experiences that have been perpetuated by systems of care, institutions, clinicians, and family members. The ultimate outcome is to achieve comfort for patients who are in pain or discomfort. The effectiveness of pain treatments depends greatly on the strength of the clinician-patient relationship; pain treatment is never about the clinician's intervention alone but about the clinician and patient (and family) working together (IOM, 2011). The IOM states explicitly, "When the clinician-patient relationship results in an authentic human connection, positive modulation of pain leads to the development of a comfort zone where caring and healing live. This creates a good partnership with the health care system, effects some resolution of internal intensifiers, honors the patient's pain experience, and impacts the person's wellbeing" (p. 22).

Application

Figure A.2 applies the therapeutic practices to pain- and comfort-specific competencies.

Attuning
The practice of being present in the moment and tuning in to an individual or situation.

Notices verbal and nonverbal cues indicating pain and discomfort and responds appropriately.

Notices verbal and nonverbal cues indicating anxiety or distress and responds appropriately.

Is aware of own beliefs and values about individuals with pain and is able to discern how that impacts own behavior in rendering pain and comfort care.

Conveys a sturdy, compassionate, and nonjudgmental presence.

Establishes a foundation for a trusting relationship.

Notices the energy and situation in the room upon entering.

Notices own energy, proximity, and pace of communication. Self-regulates as needed.

Connects with the patient/family with a focus on their state of being and pain and comfort (physical, emotional, mental, spiritual).

Conveys a genuine interest in the person's experience of comfort along with assessment of pain.

Wondering

The practice of being genuinely interested in the person. It requires an openhearted curiosity about what can be learned about this unique individual, while intentionally suspending assumptions and judgment.

Demonstrates openness and interest in the person's perception of pain/comfort.

Asks open-ended questions about their experience with comfort/pain relief in the past. Honors person's story.

Stays open and curious to new data and information from and about the person.

Avoids assumptions and consciously suspends judgments.

Following

The practice of listening to and focusing on what an individual is teaching us about what matters most to them and allowing that information to guide our interactions with the person. It requires consciously suspending our own agenda.

Listens closely to the patient's and family's concerns.

Collaborates with the involved patient/family as partners in their own care.

Listens to what is said and notices what is not said regarding pain and comfort.

Collaborates to create a plan of care that alleviates pain and promotes comfort.

Builds a sense of safety and trust by remembering specific patient and family needs and requests and including them in the plan of care.

Refrains from interrupting, correcting, rushing to fix, advise, or correct prior to hearing the person's perspective.

Clarifies and inquires about areas of concern and/or disagreement.

Notices cues to offer touch as appropriate.

Holding

The practice of intentionally creating a safe haven to protect the safety and dignity of an individual.

Practices with love and understanding.

Communicates a belief in the patient's perception of pain and suffering.

Provides care with the knowledge that we as humans seek a comfort state, and therefore actively differentiates between comfort-seeking and drug-seeking behaviors.

Remembers that each person has a unique backstory that will affect her interactions and perception of pain/comfort needs.

Recognizes that unresolved pain compromises a person's dignity and must be consistently attended to.

Initiates a pain consultation if pain and comfort needs are outside the scope of the practice area.

Communicates information about the patient/family to the rest of the health care team in respectful terms.

Avoids derogatory labels that may bias self or others against the patient.

Provides care alternatives that allow the person to participate in care decisions and accept the person's right to refuse.

Participates in and encourages consistent and visible teamwork to safeguard the wellbeing and comfort of the patient and family.

Remains a steady presence even in the face of strong emotions and crisis.

Recognizes anger as an expression of fear and distress and takes action to alleviate distress and promote comfort.

Figure A.2: See Me as a Person Therapeutic Practices: Core Competencies Applied to Pain and Comfort Care

Appendix B

See Me as a Person Therapeutic Practices: Core Competencies Applied to Teams

Mary Koloroutis

> **Attuning**
> *The practice of being present in the moment and tuning in to team members.*

Connects with team members with an interest in their state of being.

Takes in and observes team members' verbal and nonverbal cues and expressions.

Tunes in to the energy in the room including one's own energy, proximity, pace of communication, and impact on the whole group.

Communicates acceptance and respect for team members through listening, spoken words, and body language.

Gives focused attention to team members and seeks to include every voice.

Recognizes the potential for systems and processes to interfere with team relationships and takes appropriate action to remove barriers to human connection.

Notices verbal and nonverbal cues indicating anxiety or distress and responds appropriately.

Conveys openness, transparency, and interest in members of the team.

Conveys a positive and engaged presence on the team even in the face of rapid change and crisis.

Accepts responsibility for relationships with all team members.

Wondering

The practice of being genuinely interested in team members, including what each person can contribute. It requires an openhearted curiosity about what can be learned from each individual, while intentionally suspending assumptions and judgment.

Conveys genuine interest in all team members as people.

Asks open-ended questions.

Suspends own agenda as appropriate and seeks to learn the opinions of others.

Communicates an openness and desire to listen and learn from colleagues in all disciplines and services.

Conveys respect for human diversity and individual circumstances.

Avoids assumptions and consciously suspends judgments.

Is aware of potential for personal bias and refrains from stereotyping, labeling, or diminishing team members.

Stays open to and curious about new information about team members.

Remembers that each person has a unique backstory that affects his or her interactions and responses to work situations.

Challenges oneself and one's own mindset to reflect the complete situation and experience of all involved.

Following

The practice of listening to and focusing on what a team member is teaching us about what matters most to them and allowing that information to guide our interactions with the person.

Collaborates with team members.

Listens with an interest to the unique perspective of team members.

Provides sufficient time and attention for colleagues to share what is on their minds.

Refrains from interrupting, correcting, or rushing to fix prior to hearing another person's perspective.

Notices and responds to individual's cues and/or expressed preferences regarding proximity, eye contact, touch, preferred name, etc.

Clarifies and seeks to resolve areas of concern and/or disagreement.

Identifies and resolves conflicts with direct, open, and honest communication.

Builds trust by remembering specific team member needs and requests.

Holding
The practice of intentionally creating psychological safety within the team by demonstrating respect and caring and supporting conversational turn-taking.

Conveys a fundamental regard for the dignity of all team members.

Acts with integrity by following through on all commitments.

Asks for help when necessary and offers help readily.

Communicates information to the team in respectful terms and language.

Avoids derogatory labels or descriptors that may diminish other team members.

Shares information proactively so team members work well together toward a common goal.

Participates in and encourages consistent and visible teamwork for optimal patient care.

Appendix C

Role Clarity Matrix for People-Related Functions

Donna Wright and Brett Long

People-Related Function	Who has primary oversight for this process in your organization?	Who has secondary oversight for this process in your organization?
Compensation		
Benefits		
Recruitment		
Hiring		
Leadership development		
Change management/project management		
Job descriptions		
Performance evaluation		
Formal coaching and development		

People-Related Function	Who has primary oversight for this process in your organization?	Who has secondary oversight for this process in your organization?
Mandatory education/ compliance training		
Compliance tracking		
Purchasing tracking systems		
Departmental new employee orientation		
Organization new employee orientation		
New leader orientation		
Ongoing education		
New equipment training and education		

APPENDIX D

Impact of Relationship-Based Care as Reported by Organization Leaders

CATHERINE PERRIZO AND SUSAN WESSEL

Measure	Results with RBC	Organization
Patient experience/ satisfaction	Received HealthGrades Patient Safety Excellence Award, with patient safety indicators in top 5% of nation's hospitals.	Crittenton Hospital Medical Center
	Patient falls decreased 33% after RBC implementation, on track to reach goal of zero falls.	Texas Health Center for Diagnostics and Surgery, Dallas
	Reduced ventilator-associated pneumonias and central line-associated bloodstream infections, measured by NDNQI survey.	A South Dakota health system

Measure	Results with RBC	Organization
Patient experience/ satisfaction (Continued)	Patient satisfaction with response to call lights rose from 47th percentile before RBC to 91st percentile after RBC.	A Chicago area hospital
	Patient satisfaction rose from 7% at start of RBC to 83% after two years, 99% after three years.	Crittenton Hospital Medical Center
	Overall satisfaction/quality rating up 22% after RBC.	A Midwest VA medical center
	Inpatient satisfaction scores 14% higher than national scores after implementing RBC.	A Midwest VA medical center
	Environmental services "Room Cleanliness" question on patient survey trending above CMS Hospital Compare Database average three months after implementing RBC; scores continue to improve.	Mississippi Baptist Health System
	All nine HCAHPS indicators exceed CMS average after RBC implementation; five of nine exceed 90th percentile.	Mississippi Baptist Health System
	Birth center's HCAHPS patient satisfaction indicator for pain management rose 31.6%.	A Michigan hospital
	Highest patient satisfaction score ever achieved (10 basis points above national average), after RBC implementation.	New York Presbyterian Hospital/Columbia University Medical Center
	Over five years, mean scores in each of the 15 questions in nursing section of Press Ganey inpatient survey improved 2–6 points.	New York Presbyterian Hospital/Columbia University Medical Center
	In outpatient pharmacy, 94% of patients rated overall satisfaction with the service a 9 or 10 (on 10-point scale), the highest score of the last year and significantly over the benchmark.	A Midwest VA medical center
	Before RBC implementation, hospital target for patient satisfaction was 9 (on 10-point scale) with quarterly scores 8.55–8.81. During RBC training, patient satisfaction scores increased from 8.96 to 9.02. One year after implementation, scores remained greater than 9.0 (99th percentile).	St. Mary's Medical Center, Evansville, Indiana

Measure	Results with RBC	Organization
Staff engagement/ satisfaction	Two surgical units improved on the measurement "Job Enjoyment"; after RBC implementation, one went from 49.8 to 58.16, the other from 52.43 to 54.61 in one year. Units had only eight months of exposure to RBC when second measure taken and had already realized an increase in satisfaction.	Mississippi Baptist Health System
	Ranked 3rd in nation in Best Places to Work national employee survey by *Modern Healthcare*.	Texas Health Center for Diagnostics and Surgery, Dallas
	Nursing vacancy decreased to 2%.	Faxton–St. Luke's Healthcare, New York
	Employee satisfaction increased from 14th percentile to 68th percentile.	Faxton–St. Luke's Healthcare, New York
	Employee engagement rose from 3.71 to 4.23 in one year (scale of 1–5).	A Michigan health system (one department)
	Nurse satisfaction scores above both NCI and Magnet hospital benchmarks in all 9 categories.	A Midwest comprehensive cancer center
Financial performance	Employee turnover decreased from 18% before RBC to 3%.	Crittenton Hospital Medical Center
	Nurse turnover decreased from 16% to 3% with waiting list after RBC.	Crittenton Hospital Medical Center
	2 years after RBC implementation, turnover in ED is 5%; RN turnover rate in the ED has decreased from 20% to the low single digits.	A Michigan hospital
	Spending on agency nurses has decreased from $750K–$1 million/year prior to RBC to $250K and decreasing, after RBC.	Crittenton Hospital Medical Center
	Five of nine HCAHPS composites are in 90th percentile of CMS database, saving an estimated $251,636 for Value Based Purchasing reimbursement for FY 2015.	Mississippi Baptist Health System

Measure	Results with RBC	Organization
Financial performance (Continued)	Nurse turnover fell from 21.5% to 13.5% (approximately 75 full-time RNs), with cost savings of approximately $1.64 million/year.	Mississippi Baptist Health System
	Agency staffing costs dropped from $4.65 million/year to $0.	Mississippi Baptist Health System
	RN sign-on bonuses have decreased from $500 to $10,000 per position to $0 since RBC.	Mississippi Baptist Health System
	After RBC implemented, approximately $173,570 in Value Based Purchasing reimbursement was earned back, plus approximately $78,066 for even higher scores.	Mississippi Baptist Health System

APPENDIX E

Impact of Relationship-Based Care Found in the Literature

CATHERINE PERRIZO

The following table offers a small selection of the existing studies on the effectiveness and impact of RBC and/or its specific dimensions.

RBC Model Dimension	Research Study	Outcomes
Patient and Family Focus (Relationship-Based Care) • Care practices organized around the needs and priorities of patients and families. • Care is experienced when one human being connects with another. • Therapeutic relationship and four therapeutic practices. • Clinical empathy.	Winsett, R.P. & Hauck, S. (2011). Implementing Relationship-Based Care. *Journal of Nursing Administration*, 41(6), 285–290.	Decreased nurse turnover Increased patient satisfaction Increased caring behaviors with patients and team

RBC Model Dimension	Research Study	Outcomes
Patient and Family Focus (Relationship-Based Care) (Continued)	Hedges, C., Nichols, A., & Filoteo, L. (2012). Relationship-based nursing practice: Transitioning to a new care delivery model in maternity units. *Journal of Perinatal & Neonatal Nursing, 26*(1), 27–36.	Improved patient satisfaction Improved teamwork Improved patient safety
	The Schwartz Center. Building compassion into the bottom line: The role of compassionate care and patient experience in 35 US hospitals and health systems. (March 2015). Retrieved from https://ace-notebook.com/compassion-care-free-related-pdf.html	Improved health outcomes Reduced expenditures Increased patient satisfaction Better adherence to treatment Fewer malpractice claims Trust in physicians and other health care professionals Bridged differences in culture, race, and gender
	Riess, H. (2015). The impact of clinical empathy on patients and clinicians: Understanding empathy's side effects. *AJOB Neuroscience, 6*(3), 51–53, DOI:10.1080/21507740.2015.1052591	Improved patient satisfaction Improved adherence to treatment recommendations More accurate diagnoses Reduced distress Improved health outcomes Fewer medical errors and malpractice claims

RBC Model Dimension	Research Study	Outcomes
Patient and Family Focus (Relationship-Based Care) (Continued)	Cropley, S. (2012). The Relationship-Based Care Model: Evaluation of the impact on patient satisfaction, length of stay, and readmission rates. *Journal of Nursing Administration, 42(6),* 333–339.	Decreased readmission rates Decreased length of stay
	Faber, K. (2013). Relationship-Based Care in the neonatal intensive care unit. *Creative Nursing Journal, 19(4),* 214–218.	Improved patient outcomes Supported quality nursing care across the continuum of care Improvement in perceived collaboration and quality of relationships demonstrated by nursing, medical, and ancillary staff
	Woolley, J., Perkins, R., Laird, P., Palmer, J., Schitter, M. B., Tarter, K., George, M., Atkinson, G., McKinney, K., & Woolsey, M. (2012). Relationship-Based Care: Implementing a caring, healing environment. *MEDSURG Nursing, 21(3),* 179–184.	Improved HCAHPS scores for "nurses treated me with courtesy and respect"; "nurses listened to me carefully"; "nurses explained in way you understand"; and "communication with nurses" Reduction in total falls, falls with injury, and hospital-acquired pressure ulcers Improved patient satisfaction scores Increase in time nurses spent delivering patient care support Decrease in the amount of time nurses spent engaged in clinical documentation Decrease in administrative and clerical duties

RBC Model Dimension	Research Study	Outcomes
Patient and Family Focus (Relationship-Based Care) (Continued)	Wessel, S. (2012). Impact of unit practice councils on culture and outcomes. *Creative Nursing Journal, 18(4)*, 187–192.	Decreased nurse turnover Increased patient satisfaction Improved employee satisfaction Higher scores on patients recommending the hospital Reduced ventilator-associated pneumonias Reduced central line-associated bloodstream infections
	Wessel, S. (2016, September). Relationship-Based Care impact: Quality, safety, and satisfaction. *Nursing Management, 47(9)*, 17–19.	Increased patient satisfaction (top box patient experience scores) Reduced hospital-acquired infections Significant improvement in nurse job enjoyment scores Increased adherence to six safety measures Improved employee engagement Improved physician satisfaction
	McClelland, L.E. & Vogus, T.J. (2014). Compassion practices and HCAHPS: Does rewarding and supporting workplace compassion influence patient perceptions? *Health Services Research, 49(5)*, 1670–1683.	Improved clinical outcomes Increased patient satisfaction Improved patient safety Improved quality of care

RBC Model Dimension	Research Study	Outcomes
Teamwork and Interprofessional Practice • Open, honest communication • Trust and respect • Shared purpose • Diversity • Interprofessional collaboration • Care coordination	Kalisch, B.J., Curley, M., & Stefanov, S. (2007). An intervention to enhance nursing staff teamwork and engagement. *Journal of Nursing Administration, 37*(3), 77–84.	Improved clinical outcomes/patient safety Increased patient satisfaction Improved quality of care Decrease in staff turnover Decrease in vacancy rate
	Bitter, J., van Veen-Berks, E., Gooszen, H.G., & Amelsevoort, P. (2013). Multidisciplinary teamwork is an important issue to healthcare professionals. *Team Performance Management, 19*(5/6), 263–278.	Improved continuity of care Improved quality of service Improved productivity Increased collaboration
	Leonard, M.W. & Frankel, A.S. (2011). Role of effective teamwork and communication in delivering safe, high-quality care. *Mount Sinai Journal of Medicine, 78,* 820–826.	Reduction in patient mortality Decreased nursing turnover Reduction in adverse events Reduction in surgical complications Improved patient outcomes
	Manser, T. (2009). Teamwork and patient safety in dynamic domains of healthcare: A review of the literature. *The Acta Anaesthesiologica Scandinavica Foundation, 53,* 143–151.	Reduction in adverse events Reduction in surgical complications Improved quality of care Decreased lengths of hospital stay Reduction in patient mortality Improved staff wellbeing Improved quality of care Improved patient safety

RBC Model Dimension	Research Study	Outcomes
Teamwork and Interprofessional Practice (Continued)	Goh, S.C., Chan, C., & Kuziemsky, C. (2011). Teamwork, organizational learning, patient safety and job outcomes. *International Journal of Health Care Quality Assurance, 26*(5), 420–432.	Improved quality of care Improved financial results Improved patient safety
	Jones, A. & Jones, D. (2011). Improving teamwork, trust and safety: An ethnographic study of an interprofessional initiative. *Journal of Interprofessional Care,* 25, 175–181.	Improved patient safety Decreased staff sickness/absence levels Improved collegiality
	Kennedy, D.M., Fasolino, J.P., & Gullen, D.J. (2014). Improving the patient experience through provider communication skills building. *Patient Experience Journal, 1*(1), 56–60.	Improved patient satisfaction Improved quality of care
	Weng, H., Steed, J.F., Yu, S., Liu, Y., Hsu, C., Yu, T., & Chen, W. (2011). The effect of surgeon empathy and emotional intelligence on patient satisfaction. *Advancement in Health Science Education,* 16, 591–600.	Increased patient satisfaction
Care Delivery and Systems Design • Professional practice concepts • Organizational infrastructure for providing care • Maximizing resources	Sorokin, R., Riggio, J.M., Moleski, S., & Sullivan, J. (2011). Physicians-in-training attitudes on patient safety: 2003 to 2008. *Journal of Patient Safety, 7*(3), 133–138.	Improved physician–nurse teamwork Improved patient safety

RBC Model Dimension	Research Study	Outcomes
Care Delivery and Systems Design (Continued)	Goh, S.C., Chan, C., & Kuziemsky, C. (2011). Teamwork, organizational learning, patient safety and job outcomes. *International Journal of Health Care Quality Assurance*, 26(5), 420–432.	Improved patient safety Improved employee outcomes Decreased medication errors Increased nursing satisfaction Improved nurse retention Decreased nurse turnover
	Spence Laschinger, H. & Letier, M.P. (2006). The impact of nursing work environments on patient safety outcomes: The mediating role of burnout/engagement. *Journal of Nursing Administration*, 36(5), 259–267.	Improved nurse engagement Improved patient safety Improved patient care quality Decreased adverse events Decreased nurse burnout Improved nurse-sensitive patient outcomes Improved clinical outcomes
	Barsade, S. & O'Neill, O. (2014). What's love got to do with it? A longitudinal study of the culture of companionate love and employee and client outcomes in a long-term care setting. *Administrative Science Quarterly*, 59(4), 551–598.	Decreased employee absenteeism Improved teamwork Increased employee work satisfaction Increased patient satisfaction Improved patient quality of life measured in terms of dignity Improved patient relationships Improved patient mood Decreased emergency room visits
	Vital Smarts (2005). Silence kills: The seven crucial conversations® for healthcare. Vital Smarts. Retrieved from https://www.silenttreatmentstudy.com/silencekills/SilenceKills.pdf	Reduction in nurse turnover Increased employee satisfaction Increased patient safety Improved productivity

RBC Model Dimension	Research Study	Outcomes
Care Delivery and Systems Design (Continued)	Van Bogaert, P., Wouters, K., Willems, R., Mondelaers, M., & Clarke, S. (2013). Work engagement supports nurse workforce stability and quality of care: Nursing team-level analysis in psychiatric hospitals. *Journal of Psychiatric and Mental Health Nursing, 20*, 679–686.	Increased employee satisfaction Reduction in nurse turnover Improved patient outcomes
Leadership • Acting with purpose • Empowerment of staff • Removing barriers • Holding patients, families, and staff as highest priority	Spence Laschinger, H.K. & Fida, R. (2015). Linking nurses' perceptions of patient care quality to job satisfaction: The role of authentic leadership and empowering professional practice environments. *Journal of Nursing Administration, 45*(5), 276–286.	Improved nurse satisfaction Improved patient care
	Spence Laschinger, H. & Letier, M.P. (2006). The impact of nursing work environments on patient safety outcomes: The mediating role of burnout/engagement. *Journal of Nursing Administration, 36*(5), 259–267.	Decreased nurse burnout Improved nurse engagement Improved quality of care
	Yancer, D.A. (2012). Betrayed trust: Healing a broken hospital through servant leadership. *Nursing Administration Quarterly, 36*(1), 63–803	Improved hospital profitability Reduction in hospital and emergency department average length of stay, patient boarding, and ambulance diversions Improved patient satisfaction Improved quality of care

ACKNOWLEDGMENTS

We would like to acknowledge the people who helped make this book possible. A multi-authored book is a unique challenge, and we are profoundly grateful for the contribution of every author in these pages.

We would especially like to thank Rebecca Smith for her leadership in the writing of this book. She sharpened the thinking of all writers and both editors at every turn and unified the varied voices in this book. We'd also like to acknowledge the special contribution of Ann Flanagan Petry for stepping in, late in the game, as an additional developmental editor. Ann's deep knowledge of both the health care field and positive organizational development broadened and enriched our thinking and the final manuscript.

We appreciate all of the support we received from the team at Creative Health Care Management who reviewed and edited the manuscript. We are particularly grateful to Marty Lewis-Hunstiger for her meticulous editing and for the careful copyediting of Catherine Perrizo, Renee Johnson, Chris Bjork, and Kary Gillenwaters. We are grateful to Chris Bjork for his management of this project.

We also offer a special thanks to Jay Monroe for his design of this book.

ABOUT THE AUTHORS

Mary Koloroutis, MSN, RN, has been a consultant and executive leader at Creative Health Care Management (CHCM) for more than 17 years and is currently serving as CEO. Her clinical background is in oncology and maternal child health. She has served in a variety of leadership roles from clinical manager to division administrator for patient care services. Mary's work has been strongly influenced by her role as co-chair of an ethics committee in a large tertiary center. She has also served on the nursing faculties of the University of North Dakota and Metropolitan State University, focusing on management and leadership theory and application. In her 40 years in health care and academic organizations, she has worked on strategic planning and design, achieving results through leveraging the strengths and capacities of different constituencies, recruiting and developing leaders and clinical staff, and assuring high-quality care and service. She has expertise in patient- and family-centered care, medical staff relationships, and professional nursing practice.

Mary led the creation of the seminar, *Re-Igniting the Spirit of Caring*, which has influenced culture change in organizations for more than 25 years. She is co-author and editor of *Relationship-Based Care: A Model for Transforming Practice*, co-editor of the *Relationship-Based Care Field Guide*, and co-author and co-creator of the book and workshop, *See Me as a Person: Creating Therapeutic Relationships with Patients and Their Families*, as well as being the author of many scholarly articles. She is an internationally known speaker and facilitator on Relationship-Based Care, transformational leadership, therapeutic relationships, and ethics in health care. Mary's mission is to illuminate the complex and sacred nature of the work of human caring and to help create healing cultures in which all people are treated with compassion, respect, and dignity.

David Abelson, MD, has had a long and varied career in medicine, health system design, and executive leadership. David trained in general internal medicine and practiced first in private practice and then at Park Nicollet Health Services, a large integrated delivery system in metropolitan Minneapolis. In the early 1990s, he began his leadership career with clinical process improvement followed by multiple positions including Chief Medical Information Officer and Vice President of Strategic Improvement. In 2010 David became the CEO of Park Nicollet Health Services and cultivated a culture of *Head+Heart, Together.* As CEO, David was passionate about supporting healing experiences for patients and families. He led the direction of Park Nicollet to value-based payment, culminating in 2013 with Park Nicollet's merger with HealthPartners, to form an organization combining care delivery with insurance. As Senior Vice President of HealthPartners and CEO of Park Nicollet, David led a delivery system with multiple hospitals, clinics, and specialties with a combined annual revenue of $2.2 billion.

David retired in 2014. Despite retirement, he could not resist the pull of helping organizations collaborate. He is now the President of the Institute for Clinical Systems Improvement (ICSI), a collaborative of health plans and care delivery systems dedicated to improving care in Minnesota.

David publishes a regular blog, *Between Two Waves of the Sea* (www.davidabelson.net), which contains his reflections as a physician, patient, and health care CEO. He has a special interest in mindfulness and leadership.

Jayne A. Felgen, MPA, BS, RN, has immensely enjoyed serving CHCM for 20 years as a consultant, CEO, and now as President Emeritus, senior consultant, and "Chief Exuberance Officer." Jayne's greatest professional reward has always come from nurturing the growth and development of staff, managers, physicians, and executives and from inspiring them to embrace innovations in practice that benefit patients, families, and staff. Her goal is always to help people leave a legacy by hardwiring operational infrastructures such that their efforts live beyond their tenure.

From her first collaboration with the chief medical resident as a student nurse at Johns Hopkins, her 50+ year career has been defined by partnerships with clinical professionals from many disciplines, as well as service support staff in acute and ambulatory settings, from rural care environments to urban academic medical centers. She is the co-editor of the *Relationship-Based Care Field Guide* and author of I_2E_2: *Leading Lasting Change*, as well as numerous scholarly articles and book chapters.

Kary Gillenwaters, MA, OTR/L, is a client coordinator at CHCM and a facilitator of the *See Me as a Person* service line. Her first career as an addiction counselor was foundational to her view that understanding how people make meaning during health challenges is essential when partnering with them to create effective care plans. As an occupational therapist, she has provided services in independent and assisted living, memory care, home health, hospice, long-term care, and school settings. From rural to urban, from pediatrics to geriatrics, and in direct and indirect care, Kary has a passion for identifying and meeting unmet needs, often bridging mental and physical health care. Her academic activities include facilitating problem-based learning with beginning OT students. Her guiding belief in working with "challenging" people and situations is that if we are not making progress, we just don't know enough about them yet.

Gen Guanci, MEd, BSN, RN-BC, CCRN-K, is a CHCM consultant and founder and lead of the *Cultures of Excellence* service line. Gen has worked for 25 years in the Magnet®-related world. Of the organizations to which she has provided comprehensive Magnet support, 100% have achieved initial designation or redesignation. She has served as a member of the annual National Magnet® Conference Continuing Education Task Force and an item writer for the ANCC Fundamentals of Magnet Certification Exam. She founded the Bermuda Hypertensive, Cardiac and Renal Foundation and was a training officer for the Bermuda Hospitals Board, developing the first island-wide EMT and leadership development programs. She is the author of *Feel the Pull: Creating a Culture of Nursing Excellence* and of articles on environments of nursing excellence, particularly the Magnet Journey. She holds a post-masters Certificate of Advanced Graduate Studies in Organizational Development and

Leadership. The organizing principle for her consulting is partnership: "Your success is my success."

Kristen Lombard, PhD, RN, PMHCNS-BC, is a CHCM consultant and co-lead of the *Re-Igniting the Spirit of Caring* service line. She has specialized in psychiatric-mental health nursing, gerontological nursing, Relationship-Based Care, and holistic and integrative care over her 35-year career. She developed her skills in transformational leadership in her roles as consultant, clinical nurse specialist, director, nurse manager, clinician, and program developer roles in hospital, long-term care, and home care settings; private practice; and ASN/BSN/MSN education. She has expertise in teaching about Relationship-Based Care, the therapeutic relationship, circle practice, and mindfulness and integrative practices. She is an advanced practitioner of meditation and circle practice, a Certified Healing Touch practitioner, a Therapeutic Touch practitioner, and a Reiki Master. She is author or co-author of many scholarly articles and book chapters, including "The Circle Way to Authentic Leadership," "Relationship-Based Care and Meaningful Recognition: A Formula for Success in Long Term and Sub-Acute Care," and "Creating Space for Reflection: The Importance of Presence in the Teaching-Learning Process."

Brett Long, MHA, is a CHCM consultant with expertise in helping build flourishing organizations in which teams engage, find meaning, experience purpose, and celebrate amazing accomplishments. He engages emotionally intelligent leaders to improve their own, their teams', and their organizations' performance and wellbeing. With 20 years of executive leadership experience in strategy and HR roles in large health systems, he is recognized for his skill in connecting the dots from strategy to people engagement to patient engagement and fiscal health. At CHCM, he is the lead for the physician service line as well as a facilitator for *Re-Igniting the Spirit of Caring, See Me as a Person,* and *Leading an Empowered Organization.* Brett is an inspirer, mentor, and coach in driving transformational cultural change that nurtures and empowers caregivers to deliver high-quality patient care. His mission is to help all structures, processes, and people in health care to function at their full potential while remaining grounded in the reality of the current environment.

Marie Manthey, PhD (hon), MNA, FAAN, FRCN, is a consultant and President Emeritus at Creative Health Care Management. She was one of the innovators of the Primary Nursing system of care delivery, which started in one unit at the University of Minnesota and is now recognized and sought after worldwide. Marie's ability to describe key nursing practices in universal terms has helped countless organizations implement her practices through transformational change and inspirational leadership. Throughout her life in nursing, she has been motivated by her passion for the nurse-patient relationship and its potential for healing. It begins with a simple formula: Learn what supports the nurse-patient relationship and what interferes with it, then enhance what helps and minimize what hurts. She has spent her career developing and explaining Primary Nursing practices and developing and refining processes that help nurses excel and grow.

Marky Medeiros, MSN, RN, is a CHCM consultant in the *Cultures of Excellence* service line. Marky has experience both leading an organization through the Magnet Journey and partnering with organizations committed to excellence in health care through all phases of Magnet designation. Her dedicated work with structures and processes to support foundational work in organizations can be seen in the areas of staff empowerment, leadership building, shared governance implementation and enhancement, coaching and mentoring, strategic planning, and mission and vision development. Her clinical experience is in labor and delivery. She has served as adjunct faculty for a graduate nursing program focusing on the role of the nurse executive. Her focus on developing and evaluating professional practice models reflects her passion for supporting clinical staff leaders in making the connection between professional practice and their daily work.

Tara Nichols, MS, APRN, CCRN, CCNS, ACNS-BC, AGCNS-BC, is the Clinical Nurse Specialist for Pain Management at Mercy Health Saint Mary's (MHSM) in Grand Rapids, Michigan. Her 26-year career encompasses expertise in critical care nursing, pain/comfort management, and Relationship-Based Care. She has led many interprofessional teams in change initiatives, in operationalizing the implementation of RBC, and in applying caring science theory to systems of care delivery. She is currently conducting research to measure MHSM's cultural transformation from pain management to comfort care, including the relationship of clarity (self, role, and system) and of therapeutic use of self to providing holistic health care. In helping patients and families find comfort, improve function, and experience maximum safety in a painful episode in order to foster a productive life, she is always asking the questions, "What do we believe?" and, "How do our beliefs influence our behaviors?"

Catherine L. Perrizo, MBA, is contracting officer for human resources and finance at CHCM. Her mission is to support the whole organization in the work it does to improve patients' and families' experiences. Her current role includes compiling and reporting outcomes research for CHCM's Relationship-Based Care service line and facilitation for the Role Clarity and Work Alignment service line. Catherine was instrumental in transforming CHCM's support staff into a self-directed work team and loves seeing co-workers thrive in this caring, compassionate, supportive environment. Having raised her son by herself while working and earning two college degrees, she now volunteers as a life skills facilitator for the Jeremiah Program, an organization dedicated to preparing determined single mothers to excel in the workforce, readying their children to succeed in school, and reducing generational dependence on public assistance, transforming families from poverty to prosperity.

Ann Flanagan Petry, MSW, MS Positive Organizational Development, is a consultant, instructor, and writer with more than 20 years of experience in driving performance improvement in organizations. She has a clinical background in social work and palliative care and holds certifications in Emotionally Intelligent Leadership and Coaching and in Appreciative Inquiry. She has facilitated process improvement projects in many areas including physician/patient communication. Her work focuses on cultivating resilient, mindful, emotionally intelligent team members whose skills and energy improve their own, their patients', and their organizations' performance and wellbeing.

Pamela Schaid, MA, RN, PHN, CPPM, is a consultant with CHCM, transforming cultures using Relationship-Based Care, with special expertise in post-acute settings and transitions of care. She focuses on the strengths of organizations and people to enhance patient experience, employee engagement, and organizational success. She has worked in both acute care (critical care, cardiology, and oncology), and post-acute care (home care, hospice, and public health) settings, in large systems as well as free-standing community programs. She has leadership experience as a first line manager, executive director, chief operating officer, and senior director. Her experience and perspective as a family member of consumers of health care drives her passion for exploring what works best for patients and their families and how to best deliver on our promise to care for them and about them.

Rebecca Smith, BSEd, is a developmental editor and writing coach at CHCM. She feels profoundly privileged to help bring the voices of her esteemed colleagues to readers. Her previous experience with helping others share their voices includes teaching high school English in Milwaukee's inner city. She is the author of two books (*SHOULD: How Habits of Language Shape Our Lives* and *Divine Connection without Distraction: A Guide to Pure Awake Awareness*) and has collaborated with authors in bringing several other books into existence, including *Relationship-Based Care: A Model for Transforming Practice*; I_2E_2: *Leading Lasting Change*; *The RBC Field Guide*; *See Me as a Person: Creating Therapeutic Relationships with Patients and their Families;* and the *Competency Assessment Field Guide*.

Mary Griffin Strom, MSN, RN, is a CHCM consultant focusing on helping clients use Relationship-Based Care to transform their cultures as they actualize their goal of patient- and family-centered care. She is a facilitator and coach for the *Re-Igniting the Spirit of Caring, Leading an Empowered Organization*, and *See Me as a Person* curricula. Her years of experience as a clinical nurse specialist and administrator in clinical oncology, as well as her own experience as a patient receiving cancer treatment, has led to her fierce commitment to transforming health care. Working with intensivists, social workers, and medical and radiation oncology staff, she helped create a palliative care program in a community hospital, she served as a board member of a community oncology support organization, and she helped create a support group for children whose parents have breast cancer. Mary has presented many nursing and interprofessional leadership programs, and she enjoys helping health care providers reconnect to the joy and purpose of their work.

Michael Trout, MA, is president of The Infant-Parent Institute, a clinical practice, consultation, and training facility dedicated to understanding the relationship between early social experiences and how our lives form. He has decades of clinical psychology experience in the specialty of infant mental health, in which his role has been to help parents connect with their babies. It was there that he learned the principles described in this book, including drawing on the best thinking of colleagues in many allied fields. He is the co-author of *See Me as a Person: Creating Therapeutic Relationships with Patients and their Families,* and author or co-author of numerous scholarly articles and book chapters, including "The Language of Parent-Infant Interaction: A Tool in the Assessment of Jeopardized Attachment in Infancy," "Innovation by a Family Medical Practice to Provide Infant Mental Health Services," "Working with Families of Handicapped Infants and Toddlers," "Presence and Attunement in Health Care: A View from Infancy Research," and "Cultivating Mindful and Compassionate Connections."

Susan L. Wessel, MS, MBA, RN, NEA-BC, served as a consultant at CHCM for 11 years and is currently CHCM's business development leader. She enjoys mentoring others and inspiring health care organizations about the power of Relationship-Based Care and empowered leadership. She has advanced board certification in nursing administration and has served as a content expert for the American Nurses Credentialing Center in the area of nursing administration. She has filled many leadership roles, including manager, director, and vice president of patient care, and has supported both nursing and ancillary departments in inpatient, outpatient, and home care settings. She is a co-author of *Primary Nursing: Person-Centered Care Delivery System Design* and a co-editor of the *Relationship-Based Care Field Guide.* She has published numerous journal articles and has prepared many of CHCM's educational materials. Susan has served as adjunct faculty for several graduate nursing programs, helping to prepare future leaders.

Donna K. Wright, MS, RN, is a consultant and professional development specialist with CHCM. For more than two decades, Donna has worked with health care organizations to help them create effective, meaningful programs that support staff development and competency assessment for all departments. She is the author of *The Ultimate Guide to Competency*

Assessment in Health Care and *The Competency Field Guide: A Real World Guide for Implementation and Application.* Her consulting experiences have taken her to a variety of health care settings on six continents: She has worked in rural Africa, and her *Ultimate Guide* has been translated into Japanese and is being used throughout Japan. Donna is a well-known keynote speaker; she is a member and past president of the Association for Nursing Professional Development and a recipient of their "Promoting Excellence in Consultation" award.

References

Aiken, L. H., Cimiotti, J., Sloane, D. M., Smith, H. L., Flynn, L., & Neff, D. F. (2011). Effects of nurse staffing and nurse education on patient deaths in hospitals with different nurse work environments. *Medical Care, 49,* 1047-1053. doi:10.1097/MLR.0b013e3182330b6e

Akerjordet, K., & Severinsson, E. (2007). Emotional intelligence: A review of the literature with specific focus on empirical and epistemological perspectives. *Journal of Clinical Nursing, 16,* 1405-1416. doi:10.1111/j.1365-2702.2006.01749.x

Amendolair, D. (2003). Emotional intelligence: Essential for developing nurse leaders. *Nurse Leader, 1*(6), 25-27. doi:http://dx.doi.org/10.1016/j.mnl.2003.09.009

American Medical Association (AMA). (2016). *Code of medical ethics.* Retrieved from https://www.ama-assn.org/about-us/code-medical-ethics

American Nurses Association (ANA). (2015). *Code of ethics for nurses with interpretive statements.* Retrieved from http://nursingworld.org/DocumentVault/Ethics-1/Code-of-Ethics-for-Nurses.html

American Nurses Credentialing Center (ANCC). (2013). *2014 Magnet® application manual.* Silver Spring, MD: Author.

American Nurses Credentialing Center (ANCC). (2016). *Magnet® organization characteristics.* Retrieved from http://www.nursecredentialing.org/CharacteristicsMagnetOrganizations.aspx

American Occupational Therapy Association (AOTA). (2015). *Occupational therapy code of ethics.* Retrieved from https://www.aota.org/~/media/Corporate/Files/Practice/Ethics/Code-of-Ethics.pdf

Bachmann, R., & Zaheer, A. (2006). *Handbook of trust research.* Cheltenham, UK: Edward Elgar.

Baldwin, M., & Satir, V. (1987). *The use of self in therapy,* first ed. New York: Routledge.

Barsade, S. G., & O'Neill, O. (2014). What's love got to do with it: A longitudinal study of the culture of companionate love and employee and client outcomes in a long-term care setting. *Administrative Science Quarterly, 59*(4), 551-598. doi:10.1177/0001839214538636

Bartkus, V. O., & Davis, J. H. (2000). *Social capital: Reaching out, reaching in.* Cheltenham, UK: Edward Elgar.

Bartram, T., Stanton, P., Leggat, S., Casimir, G., & Fraser, B. (2007). Lost in translation: Exploring the link between HRM and performance in healthcare. *Human Resource Management, 17*(1), 21-41. doi: 10.1111/j.1748-8583.2007.00018.x

Bergum, V., & Dosseter, J. (2005). *Relational ethics: The full meaning of respect.* Hagerstown, MD: University Publishing Group.

Berwick, D. M., Nolan, T. W., & Whittington, J. (2008). The triple aim: Care, health and cost. *Health Affairs, 27*(3), 759–769. doi:10.1377/hlthaff.27.3.759

Birks, Y. F., & Watt, I. S. (2007). Emotional intelligence and patient-centred care. *Journal of the Royal Society of Medicine*, 368–374. doi:10.1258/jrsm.100.8.368

Boeing. (2014). *Statistical summary of commercial jet airplane accidents: Worldwide operations 1959–2014.* Retrieved from http://www.boeing.com/resources/ boeingdotcom/company/about_bca/pdf/statsum.pdf

Bono, J., & Judge, T. (2003) Core self-evaluations: A review of the trait and its role in job satisfaction and job performance. *European Journal of Personality, 17*(S5–S18). Retrieved from http://m.timothy-judge.com/Bono%20and%20 Judge%20EWOP%20published.pdf

Boudreaux, E. D., Francis, J. L., & Loyacono, T. (2002). Family presence during invasive procedures and resuscitations in the emergency department: A critical review and suggestions for future research. *Annals of Emergency Medicine, 40*(2), 193–205. doi:10.1067/mem.2002.124899

Boyatzis, R., Goleman, D., & McKee, A. (2002, April). Reawakening your passion for work. *Harvard Business Review.* Retrieved from https://hbr.org/2002/04/ reawakening-your-passion-for-work

Boyatzis, R., & McKee, A. (2005). *Resonant leadership: Renewing yourself and connecting with others through mindfulness, hope, and compassion.* Boston: Harvard Business School Press.

Brown, B. (2010, December). *The power of vulnerability* [Video]. Retrieved from https://www.ted.com/talks/brene_brown_on_vulnerability

Brown, B. (2013, September). *Daring greatly: How the courage to be vulnerable transforms how we live, love, and lead.* Keynote speech presented at the International Relationship-Based Care Symposium in Huron, Ohio.

Brumbaugh, B., & Sodomka, P. (2009, August). *Patient- and family-centered care—The impact on patient safety and satisfaction: A comparison study of intensive care units at an academic medical center.* Paper presented at the 4th International Conference on Patient- and Family-Centered Care: Partnerships for Quality and Safety, Philadelphia, PA.

Bryant, J. H. (2009). *Love leadership: The new way to lead in a fear-based world.* San Francisco: Jossey Bass.

Buckingham, M., & Clifton, D. (2001). *Now discover your strengths.* New York: Gallup.

Bush, H. (2011, December). Doubling down on the patient experience. *Hospitals and Health Networks.* Retrieved from http://www.hhnmag.com/articles/4353-doubling-down-on-the-patient-experience

Cacioppo, J. T., & Hawkley, L. C. (2003). Social isolation and health, with an emphasis on underlying mechanisms. *Perspectives in Biology and Medicine, 46*(3), S39–S52. doi:10.1353/pbm.2003.0063

Cadman, C., & Brewer, J. (2001). Emotional intelligence: A vital prerequisite for recruitment in nursing. *Journal of Nursing Management, 9*(6), 321-324. doi:10.1046/j.0966-0429.2001.00261.x

Caldwell, M. (2011). *Employee engagement and the transformation of the healthcare industry* [White paper]. Retrieved from https://www.towerswatson.com/en/Insights/IC-Types/Ad-hoc-Point-of-View/Perspectives/2011/Employee-Engagement-and-the-Transformation-of-the-Health-Care-Industry.

Cameron, K. S. (2003). Organizational virtuousness and performance. In J. E. Kim & S. Cameron, (Eds.) *Positive organizational scholarship: Foundations of a new discipline* (pp. 48-65). San Francisco: Berrett-Koehler.

Centers of Disease Control and Prevention. (2015). Classification of disease, functioning, and disability. Retrieved from http://www.cdc.gov/nchs/icd/icd10cm_pcs_background.htm

Charon, R. (2008). *Narrative medicine: Honoring the stories of illness.* New York: Oxford University Press.

Chambliss, D. (1996). *Beyond caring: Hospitals, nurses, and the social organization of ethics.* Chicago: University of Chicago Press.

Chesley B. "Sully" Sullenberger: Making safety a core business function [Interview]. (2013, October). *Healthcare Financial Management, 67*, 50–54.

Cherniss, C., & Goleman, D. (Eds). (2001). *The emotionally intelligent workplace: How to select for, measure and improve emotional intelligence in individuals, groups and organizations.* San Francisco: Jossey-Bass.

Clark, P. A., Drain, M., & Malone, M. P. (2003). Addressing patients' emotional and spiritual needs. *Joint Commission Journal on Quality and Safety 29*(12), 659–670. doi:10.1016/S1549-3741(03)29078-X

Classen, D. C., Resar, R., Griffin, F., Federico, F., Frankel, T., Kimmel, N., . . . James, C. (2011). Global "trigger tool" shows that adverse events in hospitals may be ten times greater than previously measured. *Health Affairs, 30*(4), 581-589. doi:10.1377/hlthaff.2011.0190

Collins, C., & Clark, K. (2003). Strategic human resource practices, top management team social networks, and firm performance: the role of human resource practices in creating organizational competitive advantage. *Academy of Management Journal 46*(6), 740–751.

Competency (2016). In *Oxford English Dictionary (OED) Online.* Retrieved from http://www.oed.com

Cooperrider, D. L., & Whitney, D. (2005). *Appreciative inquiry: A positive revolution in change.* San Francisco: Berrett-Koehler.

Cooperrider, D. L. (2008, November). The 3-Circles of the strengths revolution. *International Journal of Appreciative Inquiry*, 8-11. Retrieved from http://www.davidcooperrider.com/wp-content/uploads/2011/10/3-Circles-of-Strengths-Revolution-x.pdf

Covey, S. (2013). *The seven habits of highly effective people: Powerful lessons in personal change.* New York: Simon & Schuster.

Crowley, M. (2016, June 1). Millennials don't want fun; they want you to lead better. *LinkedIn.* Retrieved from https://www.linkedin.com/pulse/millennials-dont-want-fun-you-lead-better-mark-c-crowley

Creative Health Care Management. (2003). *Leading an empowered organization: Participant manual.* Minneapolis, MN: Author.

Creative Health Care Management. (2010). *Transforming hospital culture with Relationship-Based Care: Crittenton Hospital Medical Center brings intentional relationships to patient care and ancillary and support services.* Retrieved from https://chcm.com/wp-content/uploads/2013/04/Transforming-Hospital-Culture-with-RBC.pdf

Creative Health Care Management. (2013). Excellent patient and family experiences: Authentic connection is the solution. *Proceedings from an intensive session presented at the 2013 International Relationship-Based Care Symposium.* Retrieved from http://www.chcm.com/wp-content/uploads/2013/12/Symposium-TR-Summary-2013-11-26-FINAL.pdf

Creative Health Care Management. (2014). *Mississippi Baptist Hospital addresses the quality of all relationships resulting in significant cost savings and improved scores* [Case study]. Retrieved from https://chcm.com/outcomes/

Curry, L., Spatz , E., Cherlin, E., Thompson, J. W., Berg, D., Ting, H. H., . . . Bradley, E. H. (2011). What distinguishes top-performing hospitals in AMI mortality rates? *Annals of Internal Medicine, 154*(6), 384-390. doi:10.7326/0003-4819-154-6-201103150-00003

Davidson, J. E., Powers, K., Hedayat, K. M., Tieszen, M., Kon, A. A., Shepard, E., . . . Armstrong, D. (2007). Clinical practice guidelines for support of the family in the patient-centered intensive care unit: American College of Critical Care Medicine Task Force 2004-2005. *Critical Care Medicine, 35*(2), 605-622. doi:10.1097/01.CCM.0000254067.14607.EB

Davidson, J. E., Savidan, K. A., Barker, N., Ekno, M., Warmuth, D., & Degen De-Cort, A. (2014). Using evidence to overcome obstacles to family presence. *Critical Care Nursing Quarterly 37*(4), 407-421. doi: 10.1097/CNQ.0000000000000041

Del Canale, S., Louis, D., Maio, V., Wang, X., Rossi, G., Hojat, M., & Gonnella, J. (2012). The relationship between physician empathy and disease complications: An empirical study of primary care physicians and their diabetic patients in Parma, Italy. *Academic Medicine, 87*(9), 1243–1249. doi:10.1097/ACM.0b013e3182628fbf

Dempsey, C. (2014). Quality improvement and evidence based practice—making the connection: Reducing suffering with compassionate connected care [Presentation slides]. Retrieved from https://www.inova.org/upload/docs/For-Nurses/Nursing %20Research/Dempsey_Inova_Dec2014.pdf

Di Blasi, Z., Harkness, E., Ernst, E., Georgiu, A., & Kleijnen, A. (2001). Influence of context effects on health outcomes: A systematic review. *Lancet, 357*(9273), 757–762. doi:10.1016/S0140-6736(00)04169-6

Doyle, C., Lennox, L., & Bell, D. (2013). A systematic review of evidence on the links between patient experience and clinical safety and effectiveness. *British Medical Journal Open, 3.*e001570. doi:10.1136/bmjopen-2012-001570.

Druskat, V., &. Wolff, S. (2001, March). Building the emotional intelligence of groups. *Harvard Business Review*. Retrieved from https://hbr.org/2001/03/building-the-emotional-intelligence-of-groups

Drenkard, K. (2010). The business case for Magnet®. *Journal of Nursing Administration, 40*(6), 263-271. doi:10.1097/NNA.0b013e3181df0fd6

Duffield, C. M., Roche, M. A., Homer, C., Buchan, J., & Dimitrelis, S. (2014). A comparative review of nurse turnover rates and costs across countries. *Journal of Advanced Nursing, 70*(12), 2703-2712. doi:10.1111/jan.12483

Duhigg, C. (2016, February 25). What Google learned from its quest to build the perfect team. *The New York Times Magazine*. Retrieved from http://www.nytimes.com/2016/02/28/magazine/what-google-learned-from-its-quest-to-build-the-perfect-team.html

Dutton, R. P., Cooper, C., Jones, A., Leone, S., Kramer, M. E., & Scalea, T. M. (2003). Daily multidisciplinary rounds shorten length of stay for trauma patients. *Journal of Trauma Injury Infection and Critical Care, 55*(5), 913-919.

Edgman-Levitan, S. (2003). Healing partnerships: The importance of including family and friends. In S. B. Frampton, L. Gilpin, & P. A. Charmel (Eds.). *Putting patients first: Designing and practicing patient-centered care* (pp. 51-70). San Francisco: Jossey-Bass.

Edmundson, A. (2012). *Teaming: How organizations learn, innovate, and compete in the knowledge economy*. San Francisco: Jossey-Bass.

Ehlenbach, W. J., Hough, C. L., Crane, P. K., Haneuse, S. J., Carson, S. S., Curtis, J. R., & Larson, E. B. (2010). Association between acute care and critical illness hospitalization and cognitive function in older adults. *Journal of the American Medical Association, 303*(8), 763–770. doi:10.1001/jama.2010.167

Elam, C. (2000). Use of 'emotional intelligence' as one measure of medical school applicants' noncognitive characteristics. *Academic Medicine, 75*(5), 445-446.

Epstein, R. M, & Hundert, E. (2002). Defining and assessing professional competence. *Journal of the American Medical Association, 287*(2), 226-235. doi:10.1001/jama.287.2.226

Engel, M. (2010). *I'm here: Compassionate communication in patient care*. Orlando, FL: Phillips Press.

Engel, M. (2012). Preface. In M. Koloroutis & M. Trout, *See Me as a Person* (p. xviii). Minneapolis, MN: Creative Health Care Management.

Felgen, J. (2007). *I2E2: Leading lasting change*. Minneapolis, MN: Creative Health Care Management.

Finn, D., & Donovan, A. (2013). *PwC's nextgen: A global generational study 2013. Evolving talent strategy to match the new workforce reality.* Retreived from http://www.pwc.com/us/en/people-management/publications/nextgen-global-generational-study.html

For family members. (2016). Retrieved from http://www. hospitalelderlifeprogram.org/for-family-members/

Fractal. (n.d.). Google search definition. Retrieved from https://www.google.com/#q=fractal

Frampton, S., Gilpin, L., & Charmel, P. (Eds.). (2003). *Putting patients first: Designing and practicing patient-centered care.* San Francisco: Jossey-Bass.

Fumagalli, S., Boncinelli, L., Lo Nostro, A., Valoti, P., Baldereschi, G., Di Bari, M., . . . Marchionni, N. (2006). Reduced cardiocirculatory complications with unrestrictive visiting policy in an intensive care unit: Results from a pilot, randomized trial. *Circulation, 113*, 946–952. doi:10.1161/CIRCULATIONAHA.105.572537

Global Aviation Information Network (GAIN). (2004). *Roadmap to a just culture: Enhancing the safety environment.* Retrieved from https://flightsafety.org/files/just_culture.pdf

Gallup. (2013). *The state of the American workplace: Employee engagement insights for U.S. business leaders.* Washington, DC: Author.

Garrouste-Orgeas, M., Philippart, F., Timsit, J. F., Diaw, F., Willems, V., Tabah, A., . . . Carlet, J. (2008). Perceptions of a 24-hour visiting policy in the intensive care unit. *Critical Care Medicine, 36*(1), 30–35. doi:10.1097/01.CCM.0000295310.29099.F8

Gilligan, C. (1998). *In a different voice: Psychological theory and women's development.* Cambridge, MA: Harvard University Press.

Gittell, J. H. (2009). *High performance healthcare.* New York: McGraw-Hill.

Gittell, J. H. (2016). *Transforming relationships for high performance.* Redwood City, CA: Stanford Business Books.

Goleman, D. (1998). *Working with emotional intelligence.* New York: Bantam.

Goleman, D. (2005). *Emotional intelligence: Why it can matter more than IQ.* New York: Bantam.

Goleman, D. (2013). *Focus: The hidden driver of excellence.* New York: HarperCollins.

Goleman, D., & Boyatzis, R. (2008, September). Social intelligence and the biology of leadership. *Harvard Business Review*. Retrieved from https://hbr.org/2008/09/social-intelligence-and-the biology-of-leadership

Granek, L. (2012, May 25). When doctors grieve. *The New York Times*. Retrieved from http://www.nytimes.com/2012/05/27/opinion/sunday/when-doctors-grieve.html

Granek, L., Tozer, R., Mazzotta, P., Ramjaun, A., & Krzyzanowska, M. (2012). Nature and impact of grief over patient loss on oncologists' personal and professional lives. *Archives of Internal Medicine 172*(12), 964-966. doi:10.1001/archinternmed.2012.1426

Greenleaf, R. K. (1991). *The servant as leader.* Indianapolis, IN: Robert K. Greenleaf Center.

Griffin, S., Kinmonth, A.L., Veltman, M.V., Gillard, S., Grant, J., & Stewart, M. (2004). Effect on health-related outcomes of interventions to alter the interaction between patients and practitioners: A systematic review of trials. *Annals of Family Medicine, 2*(6), 595-608. doi:10.1370/afm.142

Guanci, G. (2016). *Feel the pull: Creating a culture of nursing excellence* (3rd ed). Minneapolis, MN: Creative Health Care Management.

Hachem, F., Canar, J., Fullum, F., Gallan , A., Hohman, S., & Johnson , C. (2014). The relationships between HCAHPS communication and discharge satisfaction. *Journal of Patient Experience, 1*(2), 71-77. Retrieved from http://pxjournal.org/journal/vol1/iss2/12/

Halm, M. A. (2005). Family presence during resuscitation: A critical review of the literature. *American Journal of Critical Care, 14*(6), 494–511. Retrieved from http://ajcc.aacnjournals.org/content/14/6/494.full.pdf

Harris, D. (2014). *10% happier: How I tamed the voice in my head, reduced stress without losing my edge, and found self-help that actually works—a true story.* New York: Harper Collins.

Hedges, C., Nichols, A., & Filoteo, L. (2012). Relationship-based nursing practice: Transitioning to a new care delivery model in maternity units. *Journal of Perinatal & Neonatal Nursing, 26*(1), 27-36. doi:10.1097/JPN.0b013e31823f0284

Helmreich, R., Merrit, A., & Wilhelm, J. (1999). The evolution of crew resource management training in commercial aviation. *International Journal of Aviation Psychology, 9*(1), 19-32. doi:10.1207/s15327108ijap0901_2

Hernandez, M. (2016). Journey to Magnet: Relationship-Based Care. Memorial Sloan Kettering LibGuides. Retrieved from http://libguides.mskcc.org/c.php?g=245177&p=1632370

hooks, b. (2000). *All about love: New visions*. New York: Harper Perennial.

How not to get sick(er) in the hospital. (2015). *Consumer Reports*. Retrieved from http://consumerhealthchoices.org/wp-content/uploads/2015/02/CRHowNotToGetSicker.pdf

Hozak, M., & Brennan, M. (2012). Using caritas as a quality improvement structure designed to maintain Magnet certification. In: J. Nelson & J. Watson eds. *Measuring caring: A compilation of international research on caritas as healing intervention*. (pp. 195-223) New York, NY: Springer Publishing.

Institute for Healthcare Improvement (IHI). (2016). *The IHI triple aim*. Retrieved from http://www.ihi.org/engage/initiatives/tripleaim/pages/default.aspx

Institute for Patient- and Family-Centered Care. (2010). *Changing hospital "visiting" policies and practices: Supporting family presence and participation* (Executive summary). Retrieved from http://www.ipfcc.org/resources/visiting.pdf.

Institute of Medicine (IOM). (2001). *Crossing the quality chasm: A new health system for the 21st century*. Retrieved from https://www.nap.edu/catalog/10027/crossing-the-quality-chasm-a-new-health-system-for-the

Institute of Medicine (IOM). (2011). *Relieving pain in America: A blueprint for transforming prevention, care, education and research*. Retrieved from https://www.nap.edu/catalog/13172/relieving-pain-in-america-a-blueprint-for-transforming-prevention-care

Isaacson, W. (2015). *Steve Jobs*. New York: Simon & Schuster.

Jensen, P. M., Trollope-Kumar, K., Waters, H., & Everson, J. (2008). Building physician resilience. *Canadian Family Physician, 54*(5), 722-729. Retrieved from https://www.ncbi.nlm.nih.gov/pmc/articles/PMC2377221/pdf/0540722.pdf

Kalanithi, P. (2016). *When breath becomes air*. New York: Random House.

Kegan, R., & Lahey, L. (2016). *An everyone culture: Becoming a deliberately developmental organization*. Boston: Harvard Business School Press.

Kelly, L. A., McHugh, M. D., & Aiken, L. H. (2011). Nurse outcomes in Magnet and non-Magnet hospitals. *Journal of Nursing Administration, 41*(10), 428-433. doi:10.1097/NNA.0b013e31822eddbc

Kelly, J. (2013). *Where night is day: The world of the ICU*. Ithaca, NY: ILR Press.

Kepes, S., & Delery, J. (2006). Designing effective HRM systems: The issue of HRM strategy. In R.J. Burke, & C.L. Cooper (Eds.), *The human resource revolution: Why putting people first matters*. Amsterdam, NL: Elsevier.

Kita, J. (2010, October). Doctors confess their fatal mistakes. *Reader's Digest*. Retrieved from http://www.rd.com/health/conditions/doctors-confess-their-fatal-mistakes/

Kohn, L. T., Corrigan, J. M., & Donaldson, M. S. (Eds.) (2000). *To err is human: Building a safer health system* (IOM Report). Retrieved from https://www.nap.edu/catalog/9728/to-err-is-human-building-a-safer-health-system

Kolcaba, K. Y. (2003). *Comfort theory and practice: A vision for holistic health care and research.* New York: Springer Publishing.

Kolcaba, K. Y. (2010). *The technical definition for comfort care.* Retrieved from http://www.thecomfortline.com/

Koloroutis, M. (Ed.) (2004). *Relationship-Based Care: A model for transforming practice.* Minneapolis, MN: Creative Health Care Management.

Koloroutis, M., & Thorstenson, T. (1999). An ethics framework for organizational change. *Nursing Administration Quarterly 23*(2), 9–18.

Koloroutis, M. (2017). *Learning from families about what they want most when their loved one needs care.* Unpublished study.

Koloroutis, M., Felgen, J., Person, C., & Wessel, S. (2007). *Relationship-Based Care field guide: Visions, strategies, tools and exemplars for transforming practice.* Minneapolis, MN: Creative Health Care Management.

Koloroutis, M., & Trout, M. (2012). *See me as a person: Creating therapeutic relationships with patients and their families.* Minneapolis, MN: Creative Health Care Management.

Koloroutis, M., & Trout, M. (2017, February 16) An evolution of the practices . . . [web log post] Retrieved from http://seemeasaperson.com/an-evolution-of-the-practices/

Kopp, D. (2013). *Therapeutic relationships: How physicians can rediscover the joy of practice while improving quality and producing safer outcomes* [White paper]. Retrieved from http://www.chcm.com/wp-content/uploads/2013/12/Dan-Kopp-Thought-Paper-2014-01-17.pdf

Labella, A. M., Merel, S. E., & Phelan, E. A. (2011). Ten ways to improve the care of elderly patients in the hospital. *Journal of Hospital Medicine, 6*(6), 351–357. doi:10.1002/jhm.900

Landrigan, C. P., Parry, G. J., Bones, C. B., Hackbarth, A. D., Goldman, D. A., & Sharek, P. J. (2010). Temporal trends in rates of patient harm resulting from medical care. *New England Journal of Medicine, 363,* 2124-2134. doi:10.1056/NEJMsa1004404

REFERENCES

Lashley, M., Neal, M., Slunt, E., Berman, L., & Hultgren, F. (1994). *Being called to care.* Albany, NY: State University of New York Press.

Lengnick-Hall, M., Lengnick-Hall, C., Andrade, L.S., & Drake, B. (2010). Strategic human resource management: The evolution of the field. *Human Resource Management: The evolution of the field, 9*(2), 64-85. doi.org/10.1016/j. hrmr.2009.01.002

Levinson, W., Roter, D. L., Mullooly, J. P., Dull, V. T., & Frankel, R. M. (1997). Physician-patient communication: The relationship with malpractice claims among primary care physicians and surgeons. *JAMA, 277*(7), 553-559. doi:10.1001/jama.1997.03540310051034

Lewandowski, L. A. (1994). Nursing grand rounds: The power to shape memories: Critical care nurses and family visiting. *Journal of Cardiovascular Nursing, 9*(1), 54–60.

Lieberman, M. D. (2013). *Social: Why our brains are wired to connect.* New York: Crown.

Lown, B. A., Rosen, J., & Marttila, J. (2011). An agenda for improving compassionate care: A survey shows about half of patients say such care is missing. *Health Affairs, 30*(9), 1772–1778. doi:10.1377/hlthaff.2011.0539

Makary, M. A., & Daniel, M. (2016). Medical error—the third leading cause of death in the US. *British Medical Journal, 353*(i2139). doi:10.1136/bmj.i2139

Manthey, M. (1980). *The practice of primary nursing.* Oxford, UK: Blackwell.

Manthey, M. (2002). *The practice of primary nursing* (2nd ed). Minneapolis, MN: Creative Health Care Management.

Manthey, M. (2007). Responsibility, authority and accountability. In Koloroutis, M., Felgen, J., Person, C., & Wessel, S. (Eds.), *Relationship-Based Care field guide: Visions, strategies, tools and exemplars for transforming practice* (pp. 486-488.) Minneapolis, MN: Creative Health Care Management.

Manser, T. (2009). Teamwork and patient safety in dynamic domains of healthcare: A review of the literature. *Acta Anaesthesiologica Scandinavica, 53*(2), 143-151. doi:10.1111/j.1399-6576.2008.01717.x

Marsh, T. (2017). Magnet initiative. *UC Davis Medical Center.* Retrieved from https://www.ucdmc.ucdavis.edu/nurse/magnet/

Mastro, K. A., Flynn, L., & Preuster, C. (2014). Patient-and family-centered care: A call to action for new knowledge and innovation. *Journal of Nursing Administration 44*(9), 446-451. doi:10.1097/NNA.0000000000000099

Maxfield, D., Grenny, J., Lavandero, R., & Groah, L. (2010). *The silent treatment study: Why safety tools and checklists aren't enough to save lives.* Retrieved from www.silenttreatmentstudy.com

Mazor, A., Alburey, A., Volini, E., Bowden, M., & Stephan, M. (2014). *The High-Impact HR operating model* [White paper.] Retrieved from https://www2. deloitte.com/content/dam/Deloitte/global/Documents/HumanCapital/ gx-hc-high-impact-hr-pov.pdf

McClure, M., & Hinshaw, A. S. (Eds.). (2002). *Magnet hospitals revisited: Attraction and retention of professional nurses.* Washington, DC: American Nurses Publishing.

McQueen, A. C. (2003). Emotional intelligence in nursing work. *Journal of Advanced Nursing, 47*(1), 101–108. doi:10.1111/j.1365-2648.2004.03069.x

Moorthy, K., Munz, Y., Adams, S., Pandey, V., & Darzi, A. (2005). A human factors analysis of technical and team skills among surgical trainees during procedural simulations in a simulated operating theatre. *Annals of Surgery, 242*(5), 631-639. doi:10.1097/01.sla.0000186298.79308.a8

Mosey, A. C. (1986). *Psychosocial components of occupational therapy.* New York: Raven Press.

Mumford, E., Schlesinger, H. J., & Glass, G. V. (1982). The effect of psychological intervention on recovery from surgery and heart attacks: An analysis of the literature. *American Journal of Public Health, 72*(2), 141-151.

National Committee for Quality Assurance (NCQA). (2016). *Patient-centered medical home recognition* [Certification guide]. Retrieved from http://www. ncqa.org/Programs/Recognition/Practices/ PatientCenteredMedicalHomePCMH.aspx

National Pharmaceutical Council. (2001). *Pain: Current understanding of assessment, management, and treatments.* Retrieved from http://www.npcnow. org/system/files/research/download/Pain-Current-Understanding-of-Assessment-Management-and-Treatments.pdf

Neff, K. (2015). *Self-compassion: The proven power of being kind to yourself.* New York: HarperCollins Publishers.

Neff, K. (2016). [website] http://self-compassion.org/

Nieva, V. F., & Sorra, J. (2003). Safety culture assessment: A tool for improving patient safety in healthcare organizations. *British Medical Journal, 12*, ii17-ii23. doi:10.1136/qhc.12.suppl_2.ii17

Noddings, N. (2003). *Caring: A relational approach to ethics and moral education* (2nd ed., updated). Berkeley, CA: University of California Press.

Nouwen, H. (1980, 2005). *In memoriam.* (p. 16). Notre Dame, IN: Ave Maria Press.

NSI Nursing Solutions, Inc. (2016). *2016 National healthcare retention & RN staffing report.* Retrieved from http://www.nsinursingsolutions.com/Files/assets/library/retention-institute/NationalHealthcareRNRetentionReport2016.pdf

Ong, L. M., de Haes, J. C., Hoos, A. M., & Lammes, F. B. (1995). Doctor-patient communication: A review of the literature. *Social Science and Medicine, 40*(7), 903-918. doi:10.1016/0277-9536(94)00155-M

Pasero, C., & McCaffery, M. (2011). *Pain assessment and pharmacologic management.* St. Louis, MO: Mosby Elsevier.

Patient safety: What is the role for Congress?: Hearing before the Committee on Health, Education, Labor, and Pensions, U. S. Senate, 107th Cong. 25 (2001) (testimony of Lucian Leape).

Peikes, D., Genevro, J., Scholle, S. H., & Torda, P. (2011, February). *The patient-centered medical home: Strategies to put patients at the center of primary care* (AHRQ Publication No. 11-0029). Retrieved from https://pcmh.ahrq.gov/page/patient-centered-medical-home-strategies-put-patients-center-primary-care

Peplau, H. E. (1991). *Interpersonal relations in nursing: A conceptual frame of reference for psychodynamic nursing.* New York: Springer Publishing.

Persky, G. (2013, September). *The impact of persistent focus and commitment: Sustainment stories.* Keynote speech presented at the International Relationship-Based Care Symposium in Huron, Ohio.

Persky, G., Felgen, J., & Nelson, J. (2012). Measuring caring in primary nursing. In J. Nelson & J. Watson (Eds)., *Measuring caring: International research on caritas as healing* (pp. 65-86). New York: Springer Publishing.

Person, C. (2004). Patient care delivery. In M. Koloroutis (Ed.), *Relationship-Based Care: A model for transforming practice* (pp. 159-182). Minneapolis, MN: Creative Health Care Management.

Piccolo, R., & Colquitt, J. (2006) Transformational leadership and job behaviors: The mediating role of core job characteristics. *Academy of Management Journal 49*(2), 327–340.

Plaas, K. (2002). Like a bunch of cattle: The patient's experience of the outpatient health care environment. In S.P. Thomas & H.R. Pollio (Eds.), *Listening to patients: A phenomenological approach to nursing research and practice* (pp. 214-251). New York: Springer Publishing.

Plsek, P. (2001). Appendix B: Redesigning health care with insights from the science of complex adaptive systems. In *Crossing the quality chasm: a new*

health system for the 21st century (IOM Report). Retrieved from https://www.
nap.edu/read/10027/chapter/13

Porges, S. (1995). Orienting in a defensive world: Mammalian modifications of
our evolutionary heritage. A polyvagal theory. *Psychophysiology, 32*(4),
301-318. doi:10.1111/j.1469-8986.1995.tb01213.x

Porges, S. (1997). Emotion: An evolutionary by-product of the neural regulation
of the autonomic nervous system. *Annals of the New York Academy of Sciences,
807,* 62-77. doi:10.1111/j.1749-6632.1997.tb51913.x

Porges, S. (1998). Love: An emergent property of the mammalian autonomic
nervous system. *Psychoneuroimmunology, 23*(8): 837-861. doi:10.1016/
S0306-4530(98)00057-2

Porges, S. (2001). The Polyvagal Theory: Phylogenetic substrates of a social
nervous system. *International Journal of Psychophysiology, 42*(2): 123-146.
doi:10.1016/S0167-8760(01)00162-3

Porges, S. (May, 2004). Neuroception: A subconscious system for detecting
threats and safety. *Zero to Three, 24*(5), 19-24.

Press Ganey Associates, Inc. (2013). *The rising tide measure: Communication with
nurses* [White paper]. Retrieved from http://images.healthcare.pressganey.
com/Web/PressGaneyAssociatesInc/Communication_With_Nurses_
May2013.pdf

Press Ganey Associates, Inc. (2016). *Performance redefined* [White paper].
Retrieved from http://www.pressganey.com/resources/white-papers
/2016-strategic-insights-performance-redefined

Rainville, P., Bao, Q. V., & Chrétien, P. (2005). Pain-related emotions modulate
experimental pain perception and autonomic responses. *Pain, 118*(3),
306-318. doi:10.1016/j.pain.2005.08.022

Rakel, D., Barrett, B., Zhang, Z., Hoeft, T., Chewning, B., Marchand, L., &
Scheder, J. (2011). Perception of empathy in the therapeutic encounter:
Effects on the common cold. *Patient Education Counseling*, 85, 390–397.
doi:10.1016/j.pec.2011.01.009

Rath, T. (2007). *Strengthsfinder 2.0.* New York: Gallup.

Rath, K. (2014). *The Power of selection and the use of talent in driving exceptional
patient experience* [White paper]. Retrieved from http://www.the
berylinstitute.org/?page=WhitePapers#white-papers-library/?page
=WhitePapers

Ray, R. L., Mitchell, C., Abel, A. L., Phillips, P., Lawson, E., Hancock, B., . . .&
Weddle, B. (2012). *The state of human capital 2012: False summit—Why the*

human capital function still has far to go (Research Report R-1501-12-RR). Retrived from http://www.mckinsey.com/business-functions/organization/our-insights/the-state-of-human-capital-2012-report

Reason, J. (1998). Achieving a safe culture: Theory and practice. *Work and Stress, 12*(3), 293-306. doi.org/10.1080/02678379808256868

Reid, R., Coleman, K., Johnson, E., Fishman, P., Hsu, C., Soman, M., . . .& Larson, E. (2010). The group medical home at year two: Cost savings, higher patient satisfaction, and less burnout for providers. *Health Affairs, 29*(5), 835–843. doi:10.1377/hlthaff.2010.0158

Richter, J. P., McAlearney, A. S., & Pennell, M. L. (2016). The influence of organizational factors on patient safety: Examining successful handoffs in health care. *Healthcare Management Review 41*, 32-41. doi:10.1097/HMR.0000000000000033

Riess, H. (2015). The impact of clinical empathy on patients and clinicians: Understanding empathy's side effects. *AJOB Neuroscience, 6*(3), 51–53. doi:10.1080/21507740.2015.1052591

Risser, D. T., Rice, M. M., Salisbury, M. L., Simon, R., Jay, G. D., & Berns, S. D. (1999). The potential for improved teamwork to reduce medical errors in the emergency department. *Annals of Emergency Medicine, 34*(3), 373–383. doi:10.1016/S0196-0644(99)70134-4

Safran, D. G., Taira, D. A., Rogers, W. H., Kosinski, M., Ware, J. E., & Tarlov, A. R. (1998). Linking primary care performance to outcomes of care. *Journal of Family Practice, 47*(3), 213-220.

Schatsky, D., & Schwartz, J. (2015). *Global human capital trends 2015: Leading in the new world of work.* [White paper.] Retrieved from https://www2.deloitte.com/content/dam/Deloitte/at/Documents/human-capital/hc-trends-2015.pdf

Senot, C., Chandrasekaran, A., & Ward, P. (2015). Role of bottom-up decision processes in improving the quality of health care delivery: A contingency perspective. *Production and Operations Management, 25*(3), 458–476. doi:10.1111/poms.12404

Shamir, B., House, R. J., & Arthur, M. (1993) The motivational effects of charismatic leadership: A self-concept based theory. *Organization Science 4*(4) 577-594. Retrieved from http://www.jstor.org/stable/2635081

Shanafelt, T. D. (2009). Enhancing meaning in work: A prescription for preventing physician burnout and promoting patient-centered care. *Journal of the American Medical Association, 302*(12),1338-1340. doi:10.1001/jama.2009.1385

Shanafelt, T. D., Balch, C. M., Bechamps, G., Russell, T., Dyrbye, L., Satele, D., . . .& Freischlag, J. (2010). Burnout and medical errors among American surgeons. *Annals of Surgery, 251*(6), 995-1000. doi:10.1097/SLA.0b013e3181bfdab3

Shattell, M., & Hogan, B. (2005). Facilitating communication: How to truly understand what patients mean. *Journal of Psychosocial Nursing and Mental Health Services, 43*(10), 29-32.

Siegel, D. (2007). *The mindful brain: Reflection and attunement in the cultivation of well-being.* New York: W.W. Norton.

Silber, J. H., Rosenbaum, P. R., McHugh, M. D., Ludwig, J. M., Smith, H. L., Niknam, B. A., . . .& Aiken, L. H. (2016). Comparison of the value of nursing work environments in hospitals across different levels of patient risk. *JAMA Surgery, 151*(6), 527-536. doi:10.1001/jamasurg.2015.4908

Smith, R. (2016). *Should: How habits of language shape our lives.* Minneapolis, MN: Creative Health Care Management.

Shem, S. (1978). *The house of God.* New York: Berkley Books.

Sodomka, P. (2006, August). Engaging patients and families: A high leverage tool for health care leaders. *Hospitals and Health Networks*, 28–29.

Stewart, M., Brown, J. B., Donner, A., McWhinney, I. R., Oates, J., Weston, W. W., & Jordan, J. (2000). The impact of patient-centered care on outcomes. *Journal of Family Practice, 49*(9), 796-804. Retrieved from http://www.mdedge.com/jfponline/article/60893/impact-patient-centered-care-outcomes

Stewart, M. A. (1995). Effective physician-patient communication and health outcomes: a review. *Canadian Medical Association Journal, 152*(9), 1423–1433. Retrieved from https://www.ncbi.nlm.nih.gov/pmc/articles/PMC1337906/

Taylor, K. (1995). *The ethics of caring: Honoring the web of life in our professional healing relationships.* Santa Cruz, CA: Hanford Mead.

Taylor, R. R. (2008). *The intentional relationship: Occupational therapy and use of self.* Philadelphia: F. A. Davis Company.

Therapeutic use of self. (2003). *Miller-Keane Encyclopedia and Dictionary of Medicine, Nursing, and Allied Health* (7th ed.). Retrieved from http://medical-dictionary.thefreedictionary.com/therapeutic+use+of+self

The Schwartz Center. (March 2015). *Building compassion into the bottom line: The role of compassionate care and patient experience in 35 US hospitals and health systems.* Retrieved from https://ace-notebook.com/compassion-care-free-related-pdf.html

Thompson, H., & Ahrens, L. (2015). Identifying talent in your selection decisions. *Nurse Leader, 13*(4), 48-51. doi: http://dx.doi.org/10.1016/j.mnl.2015.05.011

Titler, M. G. (1997). Family visitation and partnership in the critical care unit. In M. Chulay & N. C. Molter (Eds.), *AACN Protocols for Practice series: Creating healing environments* (pp. 295-304). Aliso Viejo, CA: American Association of Critical Care Nurses.

U.S. Department of Health and Human Services, Agency for Healthcare Research and Quality (AHRQ). (2016, March). *Hospital survey on patient safety culture: 2016 User comparative database report* (AHRQ Publication No. 16-0021-EF). Retrieved from https://www.ahrq.gov/professionals/ quality-patient-safety/patientsafetyculture/hospital/hosp-reports.html

U.S. News & World Report announces the 2016-2017 best hospitals. (2016, August 2). Retrieved from http://www.usnews.com/info/blogs/press-room/ articles/2016-08-02/us-news-announces-the-201617-best-hospitals

Van Wagoner, K. (2013, September). *The rebirth of a caring culture: From distrust and disunity to compassion and joy.* Keynote speech presented at the International Relationship-Based Care Symposium in Huron, Ohio.

Visser, H. (n.d.). *Understanding chronic pain.* Retrieved from http://www. wholenessfc.com/Understanding_Chronic_Pain.pdf

Vonderhaar, K. (2016, July 28). Build a winning HR business partner [Infographic]. Retrieved from https://www.advisory.com/research/ hr-advancement-center/resources/posters/ build-a-winning-hr-business-partner-model

Ware, M., & McCabe, M. (2015). *The STM report: An overview of scientific and scholarly publishing.* Retrieved from http://www.stm-assoc.org/2015_02_20_ STM_Report_2015.pdf

Wharton University of Pennsylvania. (2014, April 02). *Why fostering a culture of "companionate love" in the workplace matters.* Retrieved from http://knowledge. wharton.upenn.edu/article/ fostering-culture-compassion-workplace-matters/

Watson, J. (2008). *Nursing: The Philosophy and Science of Caring* (rev. ed.), Boulder, CO: University Press of Colorado.

Wear, D., Aultman, J. M., Varley, J. D., & Zarconi, J. (2006). Making fun of patients: Medical students' perceptions and use of derogatory and cynical humor in clinical settings. *Journal of the Association of American Medical Colleges 81*(5), pp. 454-462. doi:10.1097/01.ACM.0000222277.21200.a1

Webber, S. S. (2008). Development of cognitive and affective trust in teams: A longitudinal study. *Small Group Research, 39*(6), 746-769. doi:10.1177/1046496408323569

Welty, E. (1996). Preface to *One time, one place: Mississippi in the depression: A snapshot album* (Revised edition). Jackson, MS: University Press of Mississippi.

Wessel, S. (2012). Impact of unit practice councils on culture and outcomes. *Creative Nursing, 18*(4), 187-192. doi:10.1891/1078-4535.18.4.187

Wessel, S. (2016). Impact: Quality, safety, and satisfaction. *Nursing Management, 47*(9),17-19. doi:10.1097/01.NUMA.0000491134.06473.5c

Wessel, S., & Manthey, M. (2015). *Primary nursing: Person-centered care delivery system design.* Minneapolis, MN: Creative Health Care Management.

Whyte, D. (2010). *What to remember when awakening: The disciplines of an everyday life.* [CD]. Louisville, CO: Sounds True.

Winsett, R. P., & Hauck, S. (2011). Implementing relationship-based care. *Journal of Nursing Administration, 41*(6), 285-90. doi:10.1097/NNA.0b013e31821c4787

Wolf, J. A. (2013). *Voices from the c-suite: Perspectives on the patient experience.* Dallas, TX: The Beryl Institute.

Woolley, A. W., Chabris, C. F., Pentland, A., Hashmi, N., & Malone, T. W. (2010). Evidence for a collective intelligence factor in the performance of human groups. *Science, 330*(6004), 686-688. doi:10.1126/science.1193147

Woolley, J., Perkins, R., Laird, P., Palmer, J., Schitter, M.B., Tarter, K., . . . & Woolsey, M. (2012). Relationship-Based Care: Implementing a caring, healing environment. *MedSurg Nursing, 21*(3), 179-184.

Worline, M. & Dutton, J. (2017, February, 28). Blueprints for bringing about compassion in the workplace [Web log post]. Retrieved from http://ccare.stanford.edu/uncategorized/blueprints-for-bringing-about-compassion-in-the-workplace/

Wosket, V. (1999). *The therapeutic use of self: Counselling practice, research and supervision.* New York: Routledge.

Wright, D. (2005). *The ultimate guide to competency assessment in health care* (3rd ed). Minneapolis, MN: Creative Health Care Management.

Wright, D. (2014). Competency programs. In S. Bruce (Ed.), *Core curriculum for nursing professional development* (4th ed.). (pp. 499-513). Chicago: Association for Nursing Professional Development.

Wright, D. (2015). *The competency assessment field guide: A real world guide for implementation and application.* Minneapolis, MN: Creative Health Care Management.

Wu, A. W. (2000). Medical error: the second victim. *British Medical Journal, 320,* 726. doi:10.1136/bmj.320.7237.726

York Hospital. (2012). *Organizational overview of exemplary professional practice.* Retrieved from https://content.wellspan.org/magnet/ood/ood11.pdf

Youngson, R. (2012). *Time to care: How to love your patients and your job.* Raglan, NZ: Rebelheart.

Youngson, R. (2016). *From hero to healer: Awakening the inner activist.* Raglan, NZ: Rebelheart.

Yukl, G. (2013). Leadership in organizations (8th ed.). London: Pearson Education.

Yule, S., Flin, R., Paterson-Brown, S., Maran, N., & Rowley, D. (2006). Development of a rating system for surgeons' non-technical skills. *Medical Education, 40*(11), 1098-104. doi:10.1111/j.1365-2929.2006.02610.x

Zolnierek, K. B., & DiMatteo, M. R. (2009). Physician communication and patient adherence to treatment: A meta-analysis. *Medical Care, 47*(8), 826–834. doi:10.1097/MLR.0b013e31819a5acc

INDEX

Note: Abbreviation "RBC" stands for Relationship-Based Care.

A

B

ABOUT CHCM

Creative Health Care Management (CHCM) is an internationally known consulting firm. Since 1978, CHCM has been partnering with health care organizations around the world to improve quality, safety, patient experience, staff and physician satisfaction, and financial performance by improving relationships at all levels.

Over the last four decades, CHCM consultants have given the world Relationships-Based Care (RBC), revolutionized the field of competency assessment in health care, and provided comprehensive Magnet®* preparation services to organizations all over the country. Our interprofessional consultation team has partnered with health care organizations of all sizes on five continents on everything from one-day presentations, to organizational and system-wide assessments, multi-day workshops, and multi-year RBC implementations and Magnet Journeys.

CHCM consultants have written and published award winning and best-selling books, including:

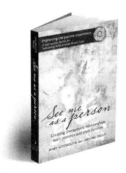

See Me as a Person: Creating Therapeutic Relationships with Patients and their Families

The Ultimate Guide to Competency Assessment

Relationship-Based Care: A Model for Transforming Practice

Competency Assessment Field Guide: A Real-World Guide to Implementation and Application

Feel the Pull: Creating a Culture of Nursing Excellence

Primary Nursing: Patient-Centered Care Delivery System Design

I_2E_2: *Leading Lasting Change*

Order CHCM's books, videos, and other products at shop.chcm.com. Volume discounts are available.

WORKSHOPS
FOR ADVANCING YOUR OWN
RELATIONSHIP-BASED CULTURE

Relationship-Based Care Practicum

The Relationship-Based Care (RBC) Leader Practicum is an immersion experience in leading a cultural change using RBC. It prepares participants to develop their own strengths as transformational leaders and to manage the details of this complex implementation.

This practical 5-day course equips RBC leaders to assemble a collaborative team of change leaders within their organizations. It is intended for a team of interdisciplinary leaders at all levels and staff who may be involved in implementation. This program provides direction for both new and experienced RBC leaders to make RBC succeed. The curriculum provides opportunity for self-discovery and reflection, networking with leaders from other organizations, strengthened relationships within your own team, and inspiration for the journey ahead.

Advancing Relationship-Based Cultures Executive Intensive

This 2-day workshop is designed for executives and strategic leaders to provide a forum to integrate and leverage Relationship-Based Care as the foundation of organizational excellence. The agenda is designed to generate discussion and strategic thinking leading to a unified vision and clear pathway for achieving the mission and goals of your organization. This experience is customized to integrate with each organization's strategic priorities and to build upon existing strengths.

Participants may include executive leaders, board members, and any other key strategic leaders.

See Me as a Person

This groundbreaking program is an impactful, cost effective, sustainable intervention for improving the patient experience.

Based on the award-winning book *See Me as a Person: Creating Therapeutic Relationships with Patients and their Families,* this two-day workshop focuses on the personal awareness, professional knowledge, and practical and repeatable skills required to see each patient as a person with his or her own unique story and response to the need for care.

This program is for all clinicians (physicians, nurses, clinical specialists, social workers, pastoral care professionals, etc.) who have contact with patients and their families. Teams of physicians, nurses, and other clinical professionals are strongly encouraged to attend together in order to deepen organizational integration of relational competence.

Re-Igniting the Spirit of Caring

Re-Igniting the Spirit of Caring (RSC) is a 3-day workshop that engages, grounds, renews, and bonds staff from all disciplines within an organization. This workshop focuses direct care providers, service support personnel, managers, and leaders on the development of three vital relationship: the clinician's or service person's relationship with self, with colleagues, and with patients and their families.

RSC is designed for leaders and staff across all roles and disciplines in all types of health care settings. RSC gathers people from diverse disciplines together so they can rediscover their common purpose and co-create a vision for what matters most in their work.

Leading an Empowered Organization

Leading an Empowered Organization (LEO) is a 3-day workshop that improves both individual and group performance in your organization. LEO participants come away with practical tools and proven strategies that make an immediate positive difference. Participants learn what it takes to be a successful leader who demonstrates purpose, authenticity, and courage.

LEO is accessible to everyone in health care. Organizations frequently send teams from various departments including nursing, respiratory therapy, plant maintenance, and human resources.

Teams that attend the program together develop the ability to hold themselves and each other accountable for modeling healthy teamwork. Over 100,000 leaders have attended this workshop worldwide.

Shared Governance Strategies that Work

Shared Governance is a model of collaboration in which decisions about practice are made by the people who will be carrying out the work, with the results of improved staff satisfaction and improved health outcomes for patients.

This practical 2-day interactive workshop provides participants with deeper clarity about what it takes to create a sustainable shared governance culture. Focus is placed on best practices; the essential structures, processes, and outcomes seen in mature shared governance cultures; and tools and resources to help both leaders and staff on the shared governance journey.

A selection of our workshops can be licensed and delivered in-house by members of your staff. We provide education, coaching, and ongoing support for your internal facilitators.

For more information about Creative Health Care Management's transformational consulting, workshops, products, and tailored organizational interventions, please call CHCM at **1.800.728.7766** or **1.952.854.9015** or visit us at **chcm.com**.